AGELESS MAN

From the Same Author

L'Andropause, cause, conséquences et remèdes

Éditions MALOINE, Paris, 1988, 1989

***

HMS WORLD Editions

El Hombre sin edad, 2016

Ageless Man, 2017

Ageless Woman, 2020

Enfermedad Androgénica en el Hombre, 2023

Androgenic Disease in Men, 2025

Ptostate Ageing Control, 2026

Georges Debled MD

AGELESS MAN

How to Cure and Prevent

Diseases of Ageing

HMS WORLD

AGELESS MAN

How to cure and prevent diseases of ageing

© Georges Debled

First edition: September 2017

Second edition: July 2020

All right reserved

HMS WORLD Editions

ISBN-13: 978-1535590143
ISBN-10: 1535590149

Contents

Author's Note 9

Medicine of Twenty-First Century 11

Part I

The Male Climacteric or Andropause

1. Sexual Ageing Announces Degeneration of All Structures of the Male Body 17
2. Male Hormones, Keys to Andropause troubles 28
3. The Castrate, a Model of Androgenic disease of andropause 35
4. Treatment with Male Hormones is an Old Concept 38
5. A Vigorous Longevity Beyond Eighty Years 47

Part II

Sexual Ageing

6. Premature Sexual Ageing 55
7. Impotence 59
8. Ejaculation Disorders 72
9. Prostate Problems 77

Part III

Diseases of Ageing

10. Diabetes and Androgenic Disease of Andropause 97
11. Male Hormones against Cholesterol 106
12. Excesses Weight and Obesity - The ideal Weight 115
13. Muscular Weakness 122
14. Arteriosclerosis or Arterial Rigidity 126
15. Anemia 137
16. Embolisms, Thromboses, Varicose Veins, and Hemorrhoids 139
17. Hypertension: Disease of the World 144
18. Coronary Disease and Heart Infarct 152
19. Stiffnesses, Limitation of the Movement, Slipped Discs, and Degenerative Joint Diseases 159
20. Fragile Bones 170
21. Skin Wrinkles 173
22. Shortness of Breath 179
23. Metamorphoses of the Silhouette 181
24. Kidney Failure 184
25. Hearing Loss and Vision Troubles 190
26. Immune Deficiency, AIDS, and Cancer 192
27. Depression 195
28. Parkinson's Disease 209
29. Dementias and Alzheimer's Disease 212
30. Stroke 227

Part IV

Revitalize your Body

31. The Anti-Ageing Hormone 233

32. Control your Ageing 239

33. Hormonal Treatment 242

Conclusion:

Ageless Man

Grow Young Again: How to Cure and Prevent Diseases of Ageing 269

Metamorphose and Rebirth of Man beyond Age Forty 272

Ageless Man 273

Bibliography 277

Author's Note

Sooner or later, starting from age forty, most men will experience various conditions and disorders: general tiredness, overweight, cardiovascular troubles, sexual problems, memory loss, irritability, and a tendency toward depression. Often, they attribute these disturbances to stress and overwork. Such concerns increase after age forty, the time of andropause.

These disorders are due to a pathological phenomenon that is the starting point of sexual ageing and diseases of ageing. I presented on this topic in Dallas in 1992.

Unfortunately, generally, that disease is not recognized. Some say it does not exist. But that disease usually begins around age forty, and sometimes earlier. This condition produces a pathological fall in the production of dihydrotestosterone, the healthy sex hormone, and sexual ageing. There is also a pathological progressive fall in testosterone that ends in deficient testosterone and diseases of ageing with time.

Sixty years ago, older adults with low testosterone were not treated because they were not detected. Life expectancy was 65 years. Older people between 60 and 80 are sometimes treated with testosterone, but their body structures have been destroyed over the last forty years. Thus, testosterone is generally contraindicated in the terminal stage of life. The misuse of testosterone explains the current therapeutic accidents and justified lawsuits in the United States.

Testosterone, in general, is contraindicated in the terminal stage of life. It is necessary to think about it forty years earlier. Moreover, the prevention of the diseases of ageing is not done by testosterone for technical reasons, as we will see later.

The subject of this book is essentially the prevention of the diseases of ageing. Sometimes, a curative effect can be achieved when a degenerative phenomenon appears. For example, a degenerative erectile dysfunction around forty or earlier can be cured if preventive treatment is correct. Another curative example is incipient sclerosis of the hand tendons, which causes finger retraction but can be cured with proper preventive treatment.

Conventional medicine for the disease is essential. Preventive medicine is a new medical profession that requires significant work before the onset of diseases of ageing. It is addressed to everyone, but especially to the younger generation.

This book explains the mechanisms of a neglected disease, the *androgenic disease of andropause.* And how to prevent sexual ageing and the pathology of ageing in men in their early stages. It is impossible to understand ageing conditions if we do not know how ageing initially occurs. Preventing diseases of ageing will allow you to live a long and healthy life.

We draw attention to diseases whose cause is not described in the medical literature. They are specific treatments for Dupuytren disease, arteriosclerosis, and Alzheimer's.

Some of the bibliographic references relate to intellectual property, allowing me to publish and date my findings in real time, as knowledge of the prevention of ageing diseases is rapidly evolving. These patents are open source.

Medicine of the Twenty-First Century

Medicine is now radically personalized to recognize the singularity of each person. It is possible to analyze the molecule encoding the genetic instructions for each organism. Each treatment can thus be made specific to the individual.

The development of cellular therapy and regenerative medicine will bring about the medical revolution of the twenty-first century: new cells, artificial or reprogrammed, will be produced to regenerate the human body or replace defective tissues or organs.

With the success of such treatments, it will be necessary to analyze and correct testosterone integrity and its metabolism in each individual.

Testosterone is essential for protein synthesis in both women and men. Consequently, it constitutes one of the bases of metabolism and is the starting point for preventing diseases due to ageing. Many recent scientific studies confirm this point.

The effects of testosterone on one's metabolism are unique to each person, man or woman, and these effects can be analyzed today. Testosterone production self-destructs over the 20 years preceding death, causing age-related diseases, so this deterioration must be corrected to avoid them. I have been addressing this topic for men since 1974, and it has not yet been contradicted and remains relevant. The lack of dihydrotestosterone and testosterone production in men produces diseases of ageing. I presented on this topic in Dallas in 1992. Beyond age sixty, two out of three men take two types of medicine, and 5 percent of sexagenarians have a form of dementia. States devote colossal sums to "looking after" diseases of ageing, which are never cured and thus constitute a bottomless financial drain.

It is necessary to understand ageing conditions and the degradation mechanisms so that men will hold their destinies in their own hands.

This book clearly shows one of the fundamental mechanisms that start the progressive deterioration of the male organism. All organs are involved. By beginning anti-ageing treatment at the onset of the first symptom, often at age forty and sometimes even earlier, it is possible to avoid age-related diseases. This book will see how the vascular deterioration responsible for Alzheimer's can be avoided. The lack of treatment for the *androgenic disease of andropause* causes entire-body degeneration in forty years, between the ages of forty and eighty. In other words, therapy to treat the androgenic disease of andropause is essential to prevent diseases of ageing.

It will take more than one or two generations for universities to begin teaching about the androgenic disease of andropause. It is too late when "medical experts" confirm a new ageing condition. Preventive treatment must begin 40 years before the disasters of old age, mainly because male hormones can currently be accurately measured.

Men over age forty and apparently in good health are actually "sick people" who ignore or are unaware of the degradation of their biochemical body structures, which leads to disease of ageing and death around age eighty, in general.

The androgenic disease of andropause is a systemic disease affecting all body structures. Today, men over eighty treated for androgenic disease of andropause on time are looking and feeling like age sixty or less and will remain ageless men for dozens of years. Until when? Nobody knows.

The average *healthy* life span in developed countries is sixty-two years, and the average life span is eighty-two years. After sixty-five, having medical insurance is impossible because insurers cover a random risk, and notthe certainty of illness or death. Indeed, the diseases of ageing (part III of this book) develop during the last twenty years of life.

Health maintenance is the medicine of the twenty-first century. The art of healing of this era is the art of preventing disease. It is based on the singular analysis of each person's biology and the particular treatments this implies: the replacement of missing hormones, the supplementation of missing vitamins and minerals, the correction of oxidative stress, and the search for carcinogenic factors.

The replacement of missing hormones must consider the androgenic disease of andropause. The biochemical understanding of this disease of ageing undermines all anti-ageing therapies. This book explains the principles of androgenic disease and andropause. It is based on clinical biochemistry, dynamic biochemistry, and molecular chemistry. These subjects are not discussed in this book, but are teaching subjects*.

The medicine of the 21st century already exists. It is evidence-based, preventive, and scientific medicine. It is the core of a new medical field that cannot be ignored since it is part of all branches of traditional medicine and concerns all physicians.

---

* The course for the SEMAL (Spanish Society of Anti-Ageing Medicine and Longevity): Barcelona, June 10, 2017: Pathologies, Diagnostics, Dynamic Biochemistry, Treatments of Men and Women in daily Anti-Ageing medical practice (In Spanish)

Course: The Androgenic Disease of Andropause and Menopause. SEMAL. III Congreso Intercontinental de Medicina Antienvejecimiento. Hotel Hilton. Panamá 17-19 de marzo 2022, (In Spanish)

Part I

The Male Climacteric

or

Andropause

The goal is not only the goal,

but the way which led there.

—*LAO-TSEU,*

Fifth to sixth century BC

1

Sexual Ageing Announces the Degeneration of All Structures of the Male Body

One day or another, sexual regression will reach all men beyond the age of forty. Unfortunately, this phenomenon can also affect young men.

Sexual ageing causes organic impotence, sterility, and disorders of ejaculation and micturition. Sexual motivation disappears, and one's general condition worsens. The end of sexual activity has been accepted less and less by men confronted with a situation in which they do not find any logical explanation.

They are unaware that, because of a insufficient information, the male hormone testosterone initially governs the structures of all proteins in the body. All organs consist of proteins, and testosterone controls their assembly. When this vital element suddenly goes missing because of Age, structures degenerate.

Testosterone also acts on the genitals by controlling their development and integrity; it is the precursor of dihydrotestosterone, the natural active sex hormone.

Reduction in the secretion of male hormones consequently provokes not only sexual ageing but also a regressive transformation of the body, which one can observe in the following ways:

• An increase in weight, with a progressive heaviness of the silhouette

• Muscular atrophy (testosterone is the muscles' food)

• Brittle bone tissue, followed by rheumatism of the shoulder, osteoarthritis of the spinal column, and so on

• Reduction of memory

Melancholia and irritability

- General tiredness, anemia
- Development of arteriosclerosis
- Varicose veins in the legs
- Hemorrhoids
- Skin that becomes thin and reddens from the sun rather than browning
- Hypertension, a consequence of arterial hardening

For everyone, the genetic clock starts the process of sexual ageing at around forty years old. Individual variations exist, which explains the later ageing of certain men, who consequently live longer. There are families in which more former members are still living, and there are others in which members die young.

This difference is probably related to the capacity of the sexual glands to secrete more or fewer hormones over time. This phenomenon also explains, among other things, the existence of centenarians.

The gene responsible for sexual ageing is not known. On the other hand, the biological characteristics and their consequences are becoming better known. Consequently, preventive medication exists, and this book aims to explain the precautionary approach.

Women's ageing has been a constant subject of study for about 50 years. Men have curiously remained conspicuously absent from these studies. However, they age too. Now that preventive medication for sexual ageing exists, it is no longer beneficial to deny it.

Certain men—and doctors—affirm that andropause is a myth or lie that does not exist. After such certainty and assertion, many men insist that the word does not exist and remain entrenched in that belief. However,

no argument denies the obviousness of andropause. It causes devastation and constitutes a new phenomenon in health and civilization.

The word "andropause" appears in a 1952 French dictionary that defines it as "the natural suspension of sexual function in older men." From the moment when a phenomenon bears a name, it exists. It is impossible to name what does not exist; however, this definition lacks precision. It is only a partial one for different reasons. First, the nuance "older" is put in, whereas it is absent in menopause. "Old" implies advanced Age and the cessation of sexual activity in men.

Consequently, finding someone older than oneself is enough to feel a certain consolation about one's sexual power. This language restriction proves that the male climacteric is accepted only with much reserve. Would the writers of the dictionary consist of younger men?

Defining andropause as "the natural cessation of sexual activity in men is correct." This degenerative phenomenon generally occurs between forty and sixty; it corresponds to menopause in women. Some will object immediately that certain men engage in sexual activity after Age sixty. But others are entirely impotent before the Age of forty. This premature impotence is much less known because the impotent ones do not speak out.

The natural cessation of men's sexual activity better defines andropause, which is not the exclusive domain of older adults. But this definition is still unsatisfactory.

In the beginning, the reduction in a man's sexual activity is not sudden. The end of sexual activity is preceded by a long period during which erections become rarer, ejaculation less generous, orgasms less intense, and libido more lukewarm. Sexual involution characterizes andropause. It extends over several years. However, it can appear in a few months.

The traditional definition also only mentions sexual cessation. But this is only one symptom among others; the most obvious is excess weight and psychological involution. Andropause is the whole of the physiological and psychological modifications accompanying the natural and progressive cessation of sexual activity in men.

Andropause characterizes the end of one's sex life, the start of which begins with puberty and, like it, extends over several years. The word *puberty* was introduced in the fourteenth century. It encompasses all physiological and psychological changes that occur during the transition from childhood to adolescence. Not until 1952 do we see a formal announcement about the end of sexual activity in older adults—andropause. At the same time, a man with andropause experiences a reduction in sexual, physical, and mental abilities.

In other words, the blossoming of sexuality accompanies the well-known transformations at puberty. The regression of sexuality, which appears with andropause, accompanies physical and psychic involution. Unfortunately, these regression phenomena are often ignored.

Women with menopause do not produce ova anymore and are inevitably sterile. On the other hand, men with andropause can even make sperm for a specific time, explaining that, after age sixty, certain men can even procreate. People use this difference primarily to deny the existence of andropause, whose definition in the French dictionary does not include the concept of fertility. However, the volume and density of sperm reach their maximum between the ages of twenty-five and thirty and decrease after that.

The same thing happens in animals. The case of Ourasi, the most famous studhorse, is a striking example. After a remarkable career in racecourses, the animal was intended for reproduction. But Ourasi, suffering from prostatic disorders, had lost his fertility.

Beyond Age sixty, fertility is possible for particular men. The case of Charlie Chaplin is famous. Even a proven case of a fertile ninety-four-year-old man [1].

A man with andropause can achieve sex from time to time, preserving individual fertility. He withdraws a certain prestige from it, but that does not mean he is as powerful as at twenty. Also, he can present all disorders of the androgenic disease of andropause, which will lead him inexorably toward unhappy old age.

Definition of the Male Climacteric and Andropause

"A different language is a different vision of life." —Federico Fellini.

Various definitions of "climacteric" do not equate with the "androgenic disease of andropause."

Climacteric

France: "Climacteric (1546) is the stage of life marking the end of the active genital period (See Menopause) in the woman and deceleration of sexual activity in man (See Andropause)." (Published in French—Dictionary Le Petit Robert).

Canada: "The period of endocrine, bodily, and psychological changes that occur with menopause. "(Published in French—French language Office of Quebec).

Spain: "The period of life which precedes and follows the extinction of the genital function." (Published in Spanish—Dictionary of the Real Academia Española).

Andropause

France: "The natural suspension of sexual function in older adults. Andropause or the male change of life. (Published in French—Le Petit Robert).

Spain: "Reduction in the genital activity in man. (Published in Spanish—Encyclopedic Dictionary Larousse).

Spain: "Age of the man whose testicular activity ceases (Published in Spanish—Dictionary of Spanish use, María Moliner).

Italy: "The period of the male life characterized by reduction and suspension of the generative capacities." (Published in Italian—

Diccionario De Mauro). This dictionary defines andropause as the period in a man's life that corresponds to his inability to procreate.

In the Anglo-Saxon world:

"Climacteric" noun: 1. a critical event or period; 2. another name for menopause; 3. the period of a man's life corresponding to menopause, chiefly characterized by diminished sexual activity (Main Collins Dictionary).

"Male menopause" is often used. Menopause means "the end of menstruation," so "male menopause" misses the point!

Various languages define "in general," a "general" phenomenon known since the middle of the sixteenth century: the suspension of sex life.

What is this phenomenon about which we are speaking? We generally talk about a disease of the ageing unknown in man: the androgenic disease of andropause. It is not solely sexual ageing. This disease announces the degeneration of the whole body.

Androgenic Disease

A weak natural androgen production produces an androgenic disease. Androgen production occurs through a series of chemical reactions, starting with the conversion of cholesterol and culminating in the synthesis of dihydrotestosterone at the receptors.

The androgenic disease begins after forty and sometimes earlier. It is due to a deficiency in the whole chain of biological androgen production. This lack leads to a defect in the manufacture of dihydrotestosterone, the last "androgen" formed and the sex hormone itself. Androgenic disease is an entity. The diagnosis is made by measuring **dihydrotestosterone,** the final metabolite[*] *in the androgen*

---

[*] Metabolite: a substance essential to the metabolism of a particular organism or to a particular metabolic process (Merriam-Webster dictionary).

production chain. Upstream metabolites are also measured in serum. Andropause is not a disease. It is a condition.

There is an androgenic disease of menopause, which is described in *Ageless Woman*.

Definition of Androgenic Disease of Andropause

Defining a new idea is not easy since there is no preliminary reference. For example, when I wrote about andropause, causes, consequences, and remedies in 1988, I described not only one new concept but a ***new disease*** [2]. Half of the booksellers in France did not know the word "andropause," even though it was registered in the dictionary. They refused this new book. Some affirmed that andropause did not exist without worrying that it is impossible to name what does not exist. I had chosen the term "andropause" because it described the principal symptom of the disease: "the suspension of sexual functions in older men" (*The Petit Robert Dictionary*). The androgenic disease of andropause describes:

The cause is reduced secretion of androgen hormones (testosterone **and dihydrotestosterone**) with age.

The sexual consequences are accompanied by or not by general disorders.

The specific treatment with mesterolone acts as dihydrotestosterone. Unfortunately, it has only existed since 1967.

In 2019, class actions in the US about the misuse of testosterone were proof that the androgenic disease of andropause is not understood. The specific treatment needs **mesterolone** and **not testosterone [3].**

The androgenic disease of andropause occurs after age forty, and sometimes earlier. Then, the production of androgen hormones (testosterone and dihydrotestosterone) decreases significantly. I proposed the following concept:

The Medical Definition of the

Androgenic Disease of Andropause

The androgenic disease of andropause is the whole of physio-pathological and psychopathological modifications that accompany the natural and progressive suspension of the sexual function in man caused by a reduction in the production of androgens [2].

Explanation of the definition:

Andropause implies reduced sexual power and problems with erections, ejaculation, and micturition (prostatic disorders). If there are no sexual disorders, there is no androgenic disease of andropause.

Reduction in the production of androgens means that the hormone dihydrotestosterone (the sex hormone) is not produced sufficiently. It results from a lack of transformation of testosterone into dihydrotestosterone. Testosterone is not a sex hormone; it can be converted to dihydrotestosterone. Consequently, the studies that do not mention dihydrotestosterone do not refer to androgenic disease of andropause.

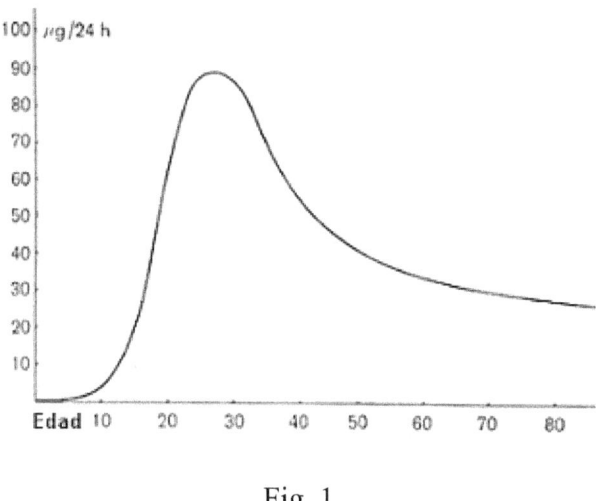

Fig. 1

Testosterone excretion decreases at various stages of life.

After Morer-Fargas [4].

The androgenic disease of andropause begins after Age forty and sometimes before. First, it starts with sexual difficulties. Then the body develops the diseases of ageing [4].

All the physio-pathological and psychopathological modifications that accompany the progressive and natural suspension of the sexual function in men are caused by the gradual reduction of testosterone secretion since this is the beginning of the androgenic disease of andropause until the final phase, which is traditional hypogonadism. If there is no symptom of sexual insufficiency, there is no androgenic disease of andropause. If no androgenic disease of andropause exists, no hormonal treatment is justified.

Since the first publication of "Andropause: cause, consequences, and remedies," the idea has spread. The scientific community today mentions the significant reduction in testosterone secretion in older adults, known as PADAM (Partial Androgen Deficiency of Ageing Men), AMS (Ageing Males' Symptoms), and LOH (Late-Onset

Hypogonadism), or, popularly, Low Testosterone. The treatment of this syndrome has been known since 1939. It is not an innovation, but it seems to spark interest in treating the weakened older adult more promptly. The important thing is to understand that the androgenic disease of andropause begins with a decrease in dihydrotestosterone production at around forty. After that, testosterone is converted to less dihydrotestosterone. Low Testosterone in older adults is the final stage of the disease. The misuse of testosterone in these cases explains the thousands of claims in the US.

Hypogonadism

General dictionaries give a broad definition.

According to the Merriam-Webster English dictionary, the medical definition of hypogonadism is "Functional incompetence of the gonads, especially in the male, with subnormal or impaired production of hormones and germ cells."

Definition of hypogonadism according to the dictionary of the Royal Spanish Academy: " Med. Defect in the function of the gonads, especially the testicles."

Hypogonadism in medical literature corresponds to the known pathological conditions treated by endocrinologists. Hypogonadism is a clinical syndrome resulting in hormone deficiency in men and women.

Primary hypogonadism is caused by gonadal (testicular or ovarian) failure.

Secondary hypogonadism results from a dysfunction in the control centers of the hypothalamus and pituitary gland. Secondary hypogonadism is rare.

Hypogonadism thus corresponds to classical pathologies with established endocrinological treatments.

Treatments for these cases of hypogonadism do not address the specific mechanism of ageing of the sex glands and their target organs. The decline in androgen production with age has constantly developed under the noses of physicians. It is called *androgenic disease*—Androgen secretion peaks around 25, and androgen production declines over the years [4].

Testosterone is not the treatment for the androgenic disease. Instead, for technical reasons, the treatment uses mesterolone (chapter 33-[7]).

There is also an *androgenic disease* of menopause, which is the subject of another book, "The Ageless Woman."

Treatment of androgenic disease in both men and women is preventive for many diseases of ageing. For example, this therapy prevents arteriosclerosis and Alzheimer's when treatment is started at the onset of these diseases.

2
Male Hormones, Keys to Andropause Troubles

Hormones are molecules secreted by an organism's glands. They convey messages or information to a target organ when released into the blood. The target cells contain receptors that trigger a reaction or signal when activated.

The primary role of hormones is to maintain the constancy of the internal environment, ensuring the organism's independence from the continually changing external world.

By mediating cell-to-cell communication, hormones integrate biochemical reactions and are essential to the harmonious development of the human body from birth to adulthood.

Other necessary ingredients include vitamins obtained from food, which contrast with hormones, which are only produced by the glands of the organism.

If hormone secretion is defective at birth, the body develops abnormally. When hormone production stops in the adult, the targets are destroyed, and the body becomes deformed.

Various glands secrete the principal hormones: the pituitary, thyroid, adrenal, pancreas, ovaries, and testicles. Each gland secretes specific substances necessary for the regulation and excellent performance of the organism. An excess or deficiency of hormonal secretion can cause specific disorders.

Testicles do not escape the law that governs all glands. But, as we will see later, their insufficient development at birth, or caused by castration, produces the castrate.

The testicles' secretion decreases gradually after the age of 25. This insufficiency causes, after forty, the appearance of all symptoms of the androgenic disease of andropause.

Testosterone, the Hormone of Long Life

The testicle produces spermatozoa and secretes androgen hormones, revealing the male sexual characteristics. They are released directly into the blood.

Androgens also have general effects necessary to the organism's construction. These effects are particularly spectacular at puberty, when the small boy transforms into a teenager and then into a fully grown man.

Testosterone is a principal hormone. Its action is observed in many organs and governs protein synthesis in all human tissues [1].

The skeletal muscle contains receptors for male hormones [2]. All individuals have a relationship between male hormone levels and muscular mass. A quite muscular man has a masculine appearance due to having higher levels of male hormones. Conversely, a man with less hormonal potential has a slender silhouette.

In pursuit of exceptional athletic performance, athletes do not hesitate to use hormones to increase their muscular mass, despite their young age and good health. Everyone remembers the "superhuman" musculature that allowed Ben Johnson to beat Carl Lewis at the Olympic Games. He was disqualified and acknowledged publicly to have taken anabolic substances.

Male hormones are particularly striking in female athletes, whose virile muscular morphology is accompanied by an almost masculine pilosity and temperament.

The International Olympic Committee classifies testosterone as a doping product; its use is prohibited among high-level athletes. The improvement of scores resulting from hormonal doping is an example of the perverse use of hormones.

The cardiac muscle is also sensitive to the effects of testosterone. In animals, testosterone administration increases the quantity of the protein responsible for the heart's contraction (actinomyosin) [3].

In 2013, a study on mice at the Department of Biochemistry, Microbiology, and Immunology of the University of Ottawa, Canada, in partnership with the Dasman Diabetes Institute in Kuwait,

showed the stimulation and differentiation of stem cells in cardiac cells due to testosterone by specifying its molecular mechanisms [4].

Bones impregnated with male hormones are solid. Testosterone acts on the skeletal structures by conferring the elasticity necessary for flexibility.

The nervous system and its sensitivity to male hormones are the objects of many studies. Receptors exist in the brain, the nerves, and the spinal cord.

Testosterone influences behaviors such as dominance, hostility, and aggression. In a population of prisoners, the plasmatic testosterone levels are higher in individuals condemned for infringements, including a concept of aggressiveness (murders, hold-ups), than in those sentenced for robbery.

Testosterone supports memory and idea generation. In addition, it determines action when its production is sufficient.

There are high levels of testosterone in the nerve cells responsible for motility and the coordination of movements. Consequently, the integrity of nerve functions depends on the proper secretion of male hormones.

The skin is known for its dependence on male hormones. For example, the prevalence of pilosity in men results from androgens, and excessive hair growth among women results from the secretion of too many male hormones.

To test the skin's quality, grip an inch between the thumb and index finger. Do not exceed one centimeter in thickness. When the fingers slacken, the skin must regain its shape instantaneously. In contrast, skin lacking male hormones remains folded for a few moments.

Red blood cell (RBC) counts increase under the influence of male hormones. Men manufacture more RBCs than women. The average red blood cell count in men is between 4.5 million and 5.5 million per cubic millimeter of blood. Men secreting sufficient male hormones have red blood cells bordering near 5.5 million.

Many studies show the favorable influence of male hormones on the body's ability to manufacture RBCs.

White blood cells (WBCs) are the immune system's guards. They contain receptors for male hormones. By stimulating WBCs, male hormones directly fight infection and cancer.

A 2012 study even showed that sex hormones stimulate telomerase activity in blood cells and, consequently, their proliferation [5].

The fluidity of the blood depends on sufficient male hormones stimulating antithrombin, a factor that improves blood flow.

Male hormones make proteins. Testosterone is the hormone of proteins and anabolism—in other words, of the organism's construction.

The liver and kidneys increase in weight after administration of male hormones. This is a normal consequence of the presence of recently incorporated proteins, which act on functional tissue.

Sugars also depend on male hormones, which act on glycogen and blood glucose.

Fats do not escape the control of androgens. A man who consults a doctor is almost always aware of his triglyceride and cholesterol levels. Still, he is usually unaware that these levels depend strictly on the secretion of male hormones.

In the blood, various fractions represent cholesterol. Those most known by the public are high-density lipoprotein (HDL) cholesterol ("good" cholesterol) and low-density lipoprotein (LDL) cholesterol ("bad" cholesterol). Testosterone favorably influences HDL cholesterol metabolism.

Testosterone regulates fat metabolism. Cholesterol and triglycerides become pathological due to a disordered hormonal secretion. Food plays a part in this disorder, but it is not the only culprit. It explains the lack of results in a man seeking a drop in blood cholesterol levels through a draconian regime.

In sum, testosterone acts on all organs and has a role in all bodily functions.

Dihydrotestosterone, the Hormone of Sexual Energy

Good sexual activity is a sign of good health. Here, also, testosterone plays a vital role.

Male hormones in sufficient quantity stimulate the normal function of the penis, testicles, prostate, and seminal vesicles.

Testosterone is not a sex hormone. Instead, it is a hormonal precursor that is locally converted into the sexually active hormone dihydrotestosterone. How does this occur? Testosterone circulates in the organism, bound to carrying proteins. Those regularly release 2 percent of the total quantity of testosterone. This free testosterone penetrates the organs to do its work there. When it enters the sexual organs, it forms dihydrotestosterone.

One consequently needs proper testosterone secretion to transform into dihydrotestosterone, the sexually active derivative.

Testosterone Secretion Drops with Age

As he grows old, a man secretes fewer and fewer male hormones. As a result, levels of testosterone and dihydrotestosterone regularly decline after age 25. This concept has been known since 1981 [6].

Interpretation of testosterone levels poses difficulties. With ageing, the number of carrier proteins increases; testosterone remains bound to them and cannot be released. Although the free testosterone is biologically active, its level decreases significantly. Consequently, there is not enough testosterone to penetrate the sexual and other organs. This phenomenon initiates the organism's involution and sets in motion a vicious cycle of self-destruction that develops over time and leads to death.

In 1991, 88 publications confirmed a reduction in total testosterone in older adults [7].

The reduction in plasma testosterone with age was confirmed between 1984 and 1993 by the School of Medicine at the University of California, San Diego. The analyzed population consisted of 810 men aged 24 to 90 years. It was Rancho Bernardo's study [8].

A reduction in the plasma testosterone level with age is also confirmed by the University of Washington Medical School, Seattle, between 1987 and 1989. In this study, 1,709 men aged 40 to 70 years were studied. Among them, 1,156 were followed for seven to ten years. It is the *Massachusetts Male Ageing Study* published in 2002 [9]. Within sexual organs, dihydrotestosterone is also less produced at an older age. As a result, the levels of female hormones can rise, leading to a feminization of older men or an involution of male sexual characteristics.

The Hormonal Singularity

Epidemiological studies of blood hormone levels give a general idea of what occurs in the population: a decrease in male hormones with ageing.

The reduction of testosterone and dihydrotestosterone production is unique to each individual. Therefore, the preferred first step is to determine the individual's androgen pool. Each man is unique and has a particular hormonal profile. A complete hormonal profile analyzes the chemical precursors of androgens and their metabolites in the urine. The measurement of the amount of these metabolites over twenty-four hours allows determining whether there is a daily hormonal overload or deficiency, thereby enabling identification of the needed hormone and adjustment of therapeutic doses. The measurement of complementary parameters is also useful. All these analyses constitute the *study of the hormonal pool of androgens*.

This comprehensive analysis is very technical. However, a simple report of assaying testosterone and dihydrotestosterone in the blood is sometimes enough.

3
The Castrate, a Model of Androgenic Disease of Andropause

The absence of testosterone secretion, after ablation of testicles, produces a being at the crossing of two sexes: the castrate, in whom profound changes appear, characteristic of sexual ageing and general ageing.

Between the two world wars, Pittard described their imposing structure in a definitive study on castrates, noting the exaggerated development of arms and legs when castration is performed before puberty [1].

Castration causes profound changes in the body. The transformations differ depending on whether an operation is performed before or after puberty. Among young boys undergoing castration before puberty, skeletal growth is modified. Changes in the skeleton contribute to the castration of his incomparable stature. Arms and legs are disproportionate compared to the trunk. The cartilage of their long bones is not welded, and their growth can continue up to age forty. Upright, the castrate is a giant. Seated, he resembles a dwarf. His skull is reduced in three dimensions; the brain is small, and the face is broader on the level of the orbits. His pelvis is large, the back is not V-shaped, and his shoulders are narrow.

The castrate does not have Adam's apple; his not-ossified, small larynx gives him an infantile soprano voice of strange beauty.

All castrates present common characteristics. However, when castrated after puberty, they look like men with an androgenic andropause disease.

The genitals of the castrated do not develop. The penis remains infantile in adults. The scrotum is small and not pigmented. Seminal vesicles and prostate are rudimentary. Regression of the genitals causes impotence and the inability to ejaculate.

Castrate tends to become obese. Fats are deposited on the hips, thighs, lower abdomen, and chest. One often notes an increase in volume in centers generally atrophied in man.

The face is typical. Eyelids simulate somnolence and present fat deposits in their outer parts. Muscles that give facial mobility are infiltrated by fat and remain fixed.

The face is puffy and fatty. Eyes are sad with an extinct glance. Aspects of eunuchs remain similar throughout their lives. Thus, it is difficult to tell their ages.

The thin, delicate skin has a waxy appearance due to reduced blood circulation. In the absence of male hormones, cutaneous pigments are missing. Castrate's skin does not brown with the sun; it reddens. Wrinkles appear quickly, and the crumpled skin of an old castrate is characteristic.

Cutaneous pilosity is poor; hairs of the pubis and armpits are sometimes absent. As a result, mustaches and beards do not develop. On the other hand, eunuchs keep thin and abundant hair; they do not know baldness.

Bones, cartilage, and ligaments are fragile. The demineralization of bones causes frequent fractures. Vertebrae are packed, and the spinal column becomes deformed.

The weakness of support tissues causes sagging of the foot's arch. The feet are flat. Knees clink. Articulations are weak, prone to osteoarthritis, and deforming rheumatoid arthritis.

Muscles do not develop, even with exercise. The heart beats slowly. Castrates are chronically constipated.

The production of red blood cells is reduced by 10 percent.

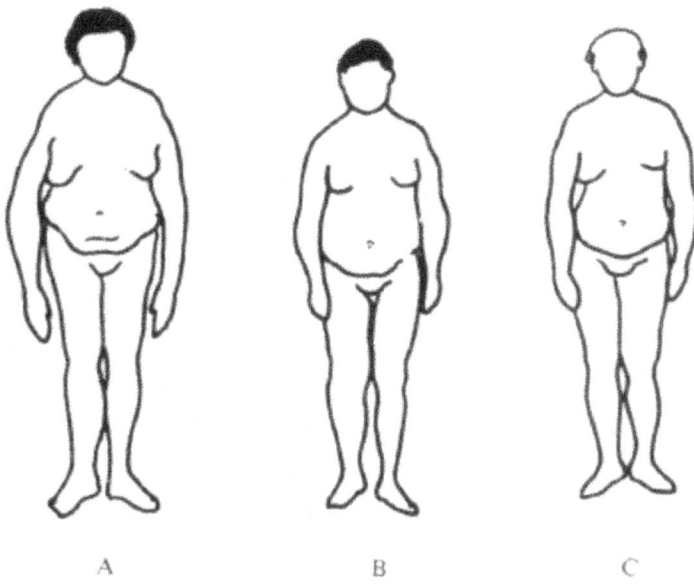

Fig. 2

A. Long bones of the castrated before puberty confer an imposing stature. At age twenty, the castrate is obese.

B. The castrato after puberty has a standard size. At age twenty, he is fat. He preserves his hair.

C. Men with andropause look castrated after puberty. Many become bald.

The brain contains specific receptors for male hormones; it is not immune to the profound effects of a lack of testosterone. As a result, the castrate is prone to depression, lacks libido, and is impotent.

4
Treatment with Male Hormones is an old Concept

The action of male hormones on the human body has been known for centuries. Aristotle, for example, had noticed the plumpness of eunuchs. At the time of Jesus Christ, the Greeks thought a substance was responsible for long life and wondered whether a relationship existed between this and sexual energy.

A lack of male hormones in animals has been known for a long time. The capon is a castrated cock. Its sexual characteristics do not develop. Its cockscomb, which is an erectile organ, remains rudimentary. The man's penis is also erectile. These organs are atrophied due to a lack of male hormones.

The beef animal is a castrated bull. Heavy and fatty, it is set to agricultural work, far from arenas and bullfighters' costumes.

In 1849, Arnold Adolph Berthold showed that the cockscomb of the capon has all its typical characteristics when the testicles are replanted in another place in the body. This experiment proves that testes secrete a substance that can act at a distance on the voice, the plumage, and the cockscomb.

Forty years later, Brown-Sequard tested on himself fresh testicular extracts from a guinea pig [1]. He described the regenerating effects and launched hormonal replacement therapy. Extracts of testicles of bulls, goats, or pigs were enthusiastically prescribed in the form of desiccated powder. But the glandular extracts have a variable composition. The lack of tangible results caused the rejection of this therapy.

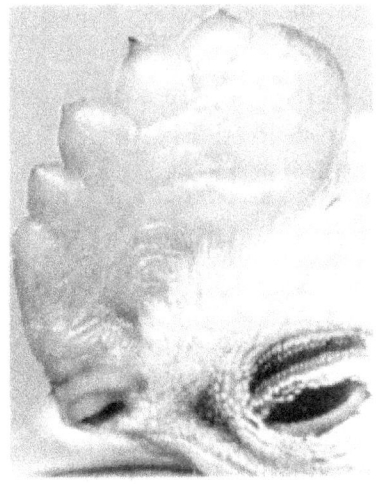 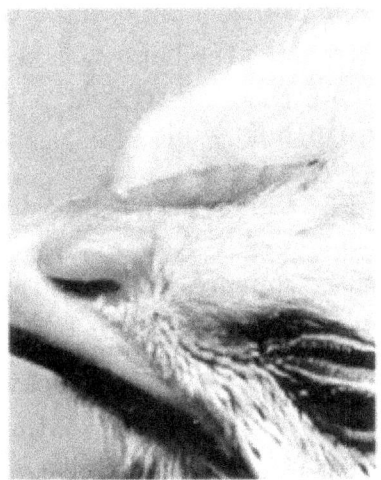

Fig. 3

A. Cockscomb with hormones   B. Cockscomb in a castrated cock

A. On the right: small, castrated cock. The cockscomb, an erectile body, is not developed (Shering document).

B. On the left: the same cock is treated with mesterolone; the cockscomb is developed and erectile (Shering document).

The studies of Voronoff remained famous. In 1930, he published his experiment with monkeys' testicular grafts, practiced on men [2]. At the same time, biologists have gradually elucidated the chemical structures of sex hormones. In addition, methods have been developed to produce synthetics.

In 1931, in seventeen thousand liters of male urine, Adolf Butenandt found fifteen milligrams of androsterone isolated in the form of crystals. This substance has an androgenic effect. A few years later, the chemical structure of androsterone was clarified as that of testosterone, the male hormone.

In 1935, Léopold Ruzicka developed the artificial synthesis of testosterone. This hormone is not very soluble. The duration of its action is short. Thus, this substance is not appropriate for hormonal treatment. In 1939, Butenandt and Ruzicka obtained the Nobel Prize in Chemistry.

In 1937, researchers modified the testosterone molecule. They obtained a soluble androgenic derivative in oils: the testosterone propionate. Injected intramuscularly, it reabsorbs slowly. Doctors from this time immediately used this hormone, of which they knew the biological properties.

In 1938, Miller, Hubert, and Hamilton [3] published a clinical study on the changes in mental activity and behavior under treatment with male hormones in two castrated patients with hypogonadism and two men suffering apparently from psychic impotence.

These patients received testosterone propionate amounts of twenty milligrams per day, or three injections per week of this same amount, compared to another series of similar patients receiving only oil injections not containing hormones.

In addition to an absence of libido and a failing erection before administering hormones, these patients were agitated and anxious. They had disturbed spirits, sometimes presenting moderate depression and occasionally severe depression.

The four patients presenting organic disorders (absence of testicles or lack of hormonal secretion) showed additional symptoms: puffs of heat comparable with those suffered by menopausal women, emotional instability characterized by sudden changes of behavior, fits of tears, periods of extreme irritability, and sometimes dark anger.

They also reported degrees of physical and mental tiredness, sometimes moderate and sometimes intense. They also complained of difficulty concentrating and low energy.

Treatment with male hormones caused essential changes, especially in the castrated, characterized by a better erection and penis sensitivity, more frequent sexual impulses, and the capacity to coincide their emotions with the sex act and the ability to embrace and intertwine.

All patients found more constant sexual activity and significant changes in their mental attitudes. The discouragement gave way to cheerfulness and even disappeared entirely in a man suffering from mental disorders.

These patients found a positive mental attitude, interest in things, and motivation in their activities. A fascinating fact is that the organic transformations occurred only among patients without testicles or a proven hormonal insufficiency. The men in this study treated with testosterone propionate were men presenting with hypogonadism.

In 1939, August A. Werner [4] described the "male climacteric" in the *Journal of the American Medical Association*. It is probably the first time this concept has been stated and described. This author had been struck by the resemblance between the symptoms of female climacteric and those of age-related changes in males. He locates the onset of the female climacteric around age 40.8, and the onset of the male climacteric between 48 and 52.

However, clinical observation had related only to two cases. The first, a fifty-year-old man, presented all the signs of female climacteric. He had healthy sexual organs. Werner prescribed ten milligrams of testosterone propionate intramuscularly, three times per week. After four weeks of treatment, subjective symptoms had sharply improved, depression was not present anymore, and he had recovered his good mood. After three months, all symptoms had disappeared. Treatment was stopped, and two months later, the signs reappeared.

The second man was forty-two years old and had undergone an inguinal hernia repair on both sides. The first operation had ended: the hernia repair had led to deterioration of the testicle, which was removed. This man had no luck because, a few years later, he underwent the same operation on the other side and lost his second testicle. Six weeks after this second operation, he became impotent and presented all signs of female climacteric.

The same hormonal treatment was undertaken, and it made all symptoms disappear. However, all signs of hormonal insufficiency reappeared after the interruption of hormonal injections.

By comparing these two cases, Werner concludes that there exists a condition comparable to the female climacteric in the fifty-year-old man that could be treated with the administration of male hormones.

Werner's patients presented a significant insufficiency in the secretion of male hormones. The first case, with apparently normal testicles, and the second case, a castrate, were men presenting with hypogonadism.

In 1944, Heller and Meyers [5] wrote "The Male Climacteric, its Symptomatology, Diagnosis, and Treatment," an article published in the *Journal of the American Medical Association*. This study summarizes many symptoms of the male climacteric:

Vasomotor symptoms: hot flashes, cold members, perspiration, palpitations, accelerated pulse, headaches.

Psychic symptoms: nervousness, irritability, insomnia, depression, negative image of oneself, antisocial tendencies, crying fits, suicidal tendencies, tingling, incapacity to concentrate.

Constitutional symptoms: muscular weakness, tiredness, pains, muscular cramps, painful articulations, lack of appetite, nausea and vomiting, pains in the belly, constipation, weight loss.

Urinary symptoms: urinary stream strength decreased, thin urinary stream, frequent urination, and difficulties urinating.

Sexual symptoms: reduction of the libido, lack of erections

The study related two groups, including thirty-eight patients. Fifteen of them presented only psychological disorders and had standard hormonal analyses. Male hormones were insufficient among twenty-three patients suffering from male climacteric, and testosterone propionate made their symptoms disappear. The authors finish their article by concluding, "Although it can appear in the thirty-year-old man, the male climacteric is rare and affects probably only a small number of men reaching an advanced age."

Men in this study, treated with testosterone propionate, were men with hypogonadism. It explains the small number of patients used by the authors of this study.

After the end of the Second World War, clinical medicine was no longer interested in the changes due to male ageing.

The androgenic disease of andropause starts with a failure to produce adequate dihydrotestosterone. Its replacement is necessary to avoid sexual ageing. There was no specific treatment for the androgenic disease of andropause before the late 1960s when mesterolone arrived on the market. Mesterolone is a mostly safe drug that mimics dihydrotestosterone (and testosterone).

In 1968, Nicholas Bruchovsky and Jean D. Wilson from Texas University, Dallas, discovered the conversion of testosterone to dihydrotestosterone in rat prostate [6]. The same year, K.M. Anderson and Shutsung Liao from the University of Chicago identified specific receptors for dihydrotestosterone in the nuclei of rat prostate cells [7]. Despite those discoveries, it is surprising that mesterolone is unknown in the United States. Therefore, in the United States, it is impossible to replace the missing hormone. The first stage of androgenic disease, andropause, is an early stage of ageing. Surprisingly, mesterolone is available worldwide—in Canada, Brazil, Mexico, the United Kingdom, China, Asia, and the European Union. My studies with mesterolone in men, which began in 1974 and have continued to the present day, have shown no side effects. Surprisingly, methyltestosterone, a toxic hormone, is available in the United States.

The diagnosis of andropause androgenic disease did not exist before 1974, when radioimmunological studies (RIA) were available in daily medical practice. Radioimmunological analyses proportioning dihydrotestosterone, testosterone, and their metabolites were consequently realisable.

The year 1974 was, for me, one of fortuity, necessity, and evidence. After studying urology for twelve years, and due to the growing number of men seeking treatment for sexual disorders, I started a consultation based on andrology. At that time, such teaching did not exist. Still, hormonal analyses in blood were performed thanks to the precision of radioimmunology, which allows hormone levels to be measured within a thousandth of a billionth of a gram (the picogram). I immediately realised that certain young men presented the same sexual disorders as older men. They were not affected by mental disorders, as was proven by exact hormonal analyses. At the same time, I was struck by the similarity in hormonal responses between young men and older adults. While comparing the results of more than a thousand cases, I concluded that andropause strikes all men beyond age forty, causing troubles with erection, ejaculation, and micturition. Then I noted that satisfied patients treated with male hormones for their sexual disorders saw their general symptoms, lack of dynamism, and depression disappear. But other diseases also went: pains of osteoarthritis, blood circulation diseases like hypertension, cardiac troubles, and anemia. This simple observation of facts enables me to affirm without hesitation that sexual ageing precedes and announces the general ageing of the human body. Furthermore, the degenerative phenomena are reversible thanks to the administration of male hormones.

Since 1974, I have prescribed mesterolone. A few years later, undecanoate testosterone enriched the possibilities of the treatment. These hormones are managed in tablets. Since 1979, dihydrotestosterone has been available as a skin gel. Today, testosterone is also available in gel form. Medical experts should know how to handle hormones to treat and prevent the consequences of androgenic disease of andropause. Indications of testosterone are not the same as those of dihydrotestosterone or mesterolone. Since 1974, I have treated thousands of men with remarkable results, and I especially noted that there is no risk of cancer with a well-proportioned hormonal treatment. These hormones have been taken continuously by many men for forty years. They are followed meticulously by doctors who have helped me for decades.

In January 1988, I published the first edition of *Andropause: Cause, Consequences, and Remedies* [8] in Paris. In 1989, I wrote a series of articles on the androgenic disease of andropause in the *Journal du médecin* in Paris [9-21].

In 1992, I published a popular book, *Au-delà de cette limite, votre ticket est toujours valable,* by Albin Michel in Paris. [22]. The same year, I presented two scientific papers devoted to the endocrine system and ageing at the International Symposium organized by the American Environmental Health Foundation in Dallas under the presidency of William J. Rea, MD: one about the male climacteric and the other about the prime causes of sexual involution [23-24]. Those papers included my experience preventing sexual and general ageing in men using male hormone treatment since 1974. This symposium drew the scientific community's attention to preventing ageing diseases through different male hormones, sparking enthusiasm among many doctors.

Since 1974, no publication has contradicted the foundation of my clinical and therapeutic descriptions of androgenic disease of andropause [8-28]. On the contrary, each day brings new scientific evidence of my basis [29].

In 2013, Professor Bansal, the chief of the department of orthopedics at the Teaching Hospital Bhairahawa in Nepal, published his 10-year study on andropause. He described this "clinical entity," confirming my definition of androgenic disease of andropause. According to this author, Nepal's population has exploded since 2007. Those over 65 are increasingly numerous. They are concerned with diseases of ageing, which constitute a "pandemic" propagated under the noses of doctors. In contrast, these diseases can benefit from a curative and preventive treatment of testosterone administration [30].

5
A Vigorous Longevity Beyond Eighty Years

Women and men constitute the most complex living structures. Their molecular combinations are the most developed and have the most elaborate brain structure among living things. Today, human beings' purely animal cerebral evolution has come to an end. The development has reached a critical stage: the spiritual transformation of humankind. This planetary phenomenon, this change without precedent in human history, is in a latent state in each of us. The great adventure has already started. Gradually, human beings release themselves from the constraints of animalism.

We remember test-tube babies—all it took to dissociate human reproduction from the act of coupling. Genetic progress will enable us to avoid the occurrence of nonviable congenital anomalies. Human reproduction will one day be without risk, both for children and mothers. The first stages of life are already scientifically reproducible, so we should be astonished by the lack of interest in the last steps.

A man lives today in a reverse mode that constitutes a dead end for humanity's future. Yet, from birth to the beginning of the androgenic disease of andropause, he generally lives in good health for forty years, the lifetime of a man in the Middle Ages.

The last forty years of a man's life are a period of senescence, or a movement toward decline and death. When, after forty, sometimes even before, sexual and reproductive regression becomes effective, it announces the arrival of successive physical and psychic degradations. Therefore, no reasonable solution can be found in the absence of hormonal prevention of ageing despite traditional medicine remedies. Given the massive deficit in health insurance and the lack of affordable health care, the solution to this crucial economic problem depends primarily on a scientific, biological approach. To age in good health is inexpensive.

Men beyond forty are prone to sexual impotence with slow movement and mentality.

During the second half of their existence, men degenerate. This degradation is regarded as impossible to stop. There is a gigantic hole in our knowledge because we are unaware of all the causes of ageing, whose consequences are well indexed and treated.

Understanding sexual regression and its degradation is the right approach toward senescence because it is possible to mitigate its effects using mesterolone. But this is addressed only to the man who reflects on himself, for the excellent reason that he must understand and participate in his treatment.

Fifty thousand years ago, man's morphology changed little. The essential changes concentrated on the human brain. This phenomenon became increasingly complex, becoming the dominant factor. The socialization of minds exists. Minds worldwide have connected, thanks to the deployment of communication resources. When an event occurs, the entire planet reacts. Tensions in the world are a striking example. This phenomenon of the brain's interconnection creates a new right: access to information. But not all are in the same boat.

There are tribes that live in the age of fire today. Certain natives of tropical areas have a life expectancy of approximately twenty years. However, whole populations still live according to the medieval mode, and have considerably reduced life expectancy. In Europe, in endangered industrial sites, communities still live as they did at the beginning of the twentieth century. In modern cities, one sees men and women defined primarily as consumers.

From the forest, via fields and cities, man became an unparalleled being, and nothing is off-limits anymore. Obsessed with having, he overlooked the road to the highest form of life: being.

But the progressive man is deep within. It is enough to boost him with information. He will then be able to understand and treat his ageing.

Failing this, what do we do? Despite the massive deployment of technological means, average longevity does not exceed eighty years; after forty years, a man slows down sexually, physically, and mentally. He is unaware that he does not secrete enough male hormones. In addition to this lack of knowledge, the disastrous effects of overeating and the total lack of muscular exercise are common.

After forty, it is initially necessary to reflect and decide to live, thanks to hormonal therapy with androgens, with a controlled diet and exercise. Men who see their symptoms disappear with hormonal treatment can diagnose their recovery from the androgenic disease of andropause by examining other untreated men and reflecting on what they were before. The man with andropause syndrome shows typical characteristics. The most obvious is the lack of shine. Conversely, the general health condition of men treated with mesterolone is surprising.

Birth and death are natural phenomena that belong to the realm of metaphysics. Between these two poles, there is life. Therefore, it is essential to know it best, overcome physical obstacles, and use its spiritual potential as much as possible. Here, industrial medicine, birthed from scientific medicine, missed the mark. Indeed, medical science aims to save and reestablish health, an absence of disease or infirmity, and a state of mental and social well-being. However, given the characteristics of industrial civilization, the medicine that has developed over the past forty years can only eliminate disease and infirmity, unaware of the state of mental and social well-being.

Does the reader know that the price of highly sophisticated apparatuses is fixed not by their manufacturing costs and a reasonable profit, but by the number of patients likely to use them and by the Social Security offices' refunds? Is wanting to escape from the natural phenomenon of death quite reasonable? Too many patients die today encumbered by machinery, even when they have reached eighty years, the limit of longevity in the industrial era. Frustrating deaths. Unworthy deaths.

Today's most common diseases are those of discomfort, whose causes are not readily apparent. They require a *comprehensive approach* to the individual, which medical experts understand. Such methods often contribute to reestablishing physical and mental well-being, essential components of health, and are not as parallel as some would like to believe.

Causes of ageing are the primary source of discomfort. They must be the subject of individual attention. What do we note? Before forty, men generally have good health and good sexual activity. Andropause marks the end of the sexual program. Gradually, ageing diseases occur—osteoarthritis, arteriosclerosis, obesity, cataracts, and skin, nail, and hair disorders. Cerebral activity is disturbed, and memory disorders appear. Migraines, gloomy moods, lack of dynamism, pusillanimity, unhappiness, and depression make their appearance up to that point unknown. These symptoms are often signs of androgenic disease of andropause.

To treat the androgenic disease of andropause—the androgenic condition of andropause—means to decrease, if not eliminate, ageing diseases so that men beyond age forty will remain in good health.

With proper treatment, mature human beings will no longer know the inevitable decrepitude that leads to death at around eighty. Men and women of fifty, sixty, and seventy years will have the aspects of their forties and be in good health. After replacing his defective parameters for twenty years, the older man of sixty consecutive years will be biologically forty.

This difference between chronological and biological age currently exists. For example, embryos are preserved in liquid nitrogen at a low temperature. When implanted in the mother, an embryo develops into a human being. An embryo frozen for 2 months results in a child whose chronological age is 11 months and whose biological age is 9 months. Thus, an embryo from several consecutive years would give rise to a being whose biological age would be only 9 months.

For the first time, humans are beginning to understand the mechanisms that govern the beginning and end of their terrestrial existence. Today, it is necessary to study the causes of ageing. The task is immense. Understanding the mechanisms of ageing will enable the full utilisation of human resources from birth to death. Men treated with mesterolone will reach their full longevity potential. After that, they will be ageless men.

Centenaries are expressions of the potential for longevity. But when they are not treated, they stop running like rabbits. With individually tailored hormonal treatment, one can imagine a human living to around 120 years old, perhaps more. The key is to get there in good health; if not, it is useless.

Specific hormones open the door to this possibility. Centenarians will not live in isolation in their rooms or without activity. We will finally be able to "die of life." Experiments show that male hormone levels are high in older adults who remain fertile and active. A publication of Nieschlag [1] confirms the existence of high rates of male hormones in older men enjoying exceptional health. They are precisely the men who could become centenarians without hormone replacement therapy.

Men treated with hormones are similar to older adults whose testicles secrete male hormones naturally and enjoy exceptional health. However, if one stops treating an older man enjoying good health thanks to hormonal replacement therapy, he will invariably degrade physically, mentally, and sexually again.

The treatment and prevention of ageing diseases increases the average longevity of the population. We will see, in twenty years, their androgenic disease of andropause, they will have been treated. In a few decades, centenarians will be in good health thanks to the proper hormonal treatment, and nobody can say today what the age septuagenarians whose biological age will be fifty years. Conscious today of limit will be.

PART II

Sexual Ageing

Sexual ageing announces general ageing.

6
Premature Sexual Ageing

A lack of male hormones causes sexual ageing, whatever the age.

In any man, testosterone secretion decreases gradually after age twenty-five. Fifteen years later, the signs of sexual ageing appear gradually, causing sexual breakdowns and ejaculation disorders.

Certain young men are not lucky; their testicles stop functioning before forty, sometimes abruptly, causing the appearance of andropause symptoms. The same phenomenon exists in young women who suffer from premature menopause.

The fetus produces primitive sexual glands. In boys, these glands migrate to the scrotum. In girls, the embryonic glands remain in the belly, making the ovaries. The testicles produce male hormones and female hormones. The ovaries produce female hormones and male hormones.

It is necessary to know about the phenomenon of premature sexual ageing because the situation of these young men with the early androgenic disease of andropause is dramatic. They do not understand what has happened to them and have poor health. Their sex lives are miserable, and their partners' repercussions are testing. It is a real-life test that feelings do not always overcome. Fortunately, there are remedies today. One quivers, however, while thinking of the generations of young men with premature sexual ageing who remained impotent due to lack of information—many committed suicides without knowing why. The causes of premature sexual ageing are multiple.

The absence, at birth, of both testicles exists. It is a rare anomaly. On the other hand, losing one or two testicles can occur during a lifetime, generally after trauma or botched surgery.

During a hernia or a genital operation, one or two testicles are castrated, causing surgical eunuchs. Fortunately, hormonal substitution treatment makes it possible to rectify this problematic situation.

There exists a whole series of factors that cause a testicle's atrophy. Sometimes it does not exceed a centimeter in diameter, and, painful, its ablation is occasionally necessary. The causes of a testicle's atrophy are multiple: traumas, irradiations, intense exposure to heat (oven, metallurgy), repeated shocks in equestrians, nicotine, alcoholism, absorption of female hormones, injury of the testicle artery, microbial infection, viral infection (mumps), malformation, or varicose veins.

Undescended Testicle

Parents are sometimes surprised not to see testicles in a child's scrotum, whereas they were there before. They are "elevator" testicles, which generally go down in the scrotum but go up high when they undergo excitation from hands or cold water.

A small muscle is inserted into the scrotum. Its sharp contraction raises the testicle. This characteristic is without gravity. The parents will be reassured by giving their child a hot bath, and the testicles will return to the right place spontaneously.

On the other hand, many testicles do not descend; they are called undescended testes (cryptorchidism).

The fetus has its testicles in its belly. In the second month of fetal life, the testes migrate to the scrotum. A certain number of testicles go down during the first year of life. For this period, there is no need to worry. The absence of testes in the scrotum beyond the first year must make us suspect undescended testicles.

The testicle is extremely sensitive to heat. The body temperature is too high, leading to the deterioration of cells that produce spermatozoa and male hormones. When the undescended testicle is retained outside the scrotum by mechanical obstacles, it is necessary to place it surgically in the scrotum at around age three or four.

An undescended testicle is often associated with a hernia. All genital areas are malformed to varying degrees, and associated anomalies must be investigated. Unfortunately, an undescended testicle will secrete generally fewer hormones after puberty, leading to premature sexual ageing. A diagnosis will be made as soon as possible to promptly replace the missing hormones.

Varicose Veins in Testicles

The testicle is connected to the belly by a cord. An artery distributes blood to the testicle, and several veins bring blood toward the general circulation. There is a duct for the emission of spermatozoa.

Dilation of these veins is not uncommon. It is caused by a backward flow of blood (instead of going up in the belly, blood returns toward the testicle; blood circulation is reversed).

In the beginning, the veins of the spermatic cord dilate. With time, the total loss of elasticity of the venous walls leads to the formation of a soft tumor above the testicle. A varicose tumor, caused by permanent dilation of the veins, is called a varicocele.

The varicocele generally appears on the scrotum's left side. However, it is not rare on the right side. It seems like a small, vermiculated package above the testicle. The palpation of this abnormal package gives the impression of macaroni under the skin. In addition, venous wall distension can cause pain.

A simple test can confirm the presence of varicose veins. If you present a small tumefaction above the testicle, lie down. The abnormal package disappears; the macaroni is not noticeable. However, they appear again when you are raised.

The varicose veins of the spermatic cord cause the atrophy of the testicle because blood circulates with difficulty. As a result, the The varicose veins of the spermatic cord cause the atrophy of the testicle because blood circulates with difficulty. As a result, the secretion of male hormones is disturbed, followed by ejaculation, erection, and urination disorders. These chronic symptoms often go back for several years and are accentuated with time.

The varicose veins of the testicle are a frequent cause of male sterility. The disturbance of hormonal secretion is less known; however, it has been confirmed by clinical studies for over forty years. The reduction in hormonal secretion in carriers of varicose veins is significant [1].

The deceleration of blood circulation in the varicose testicle causes inadequate oxygenation of the cells, destroying those that produce spermatozoids and those that secrete male hormones.

Impotence comes not only from the disordered hormonal secretion but also from the blood escape during erection. Instead of being imprisoned in the penis in an erection, blood leaks into the varicose veins, particularly the veins of the penis communicating with the venous network of the testicles.

The treatment of the varicose veins of the testicle is surgical. Several techniques exist, but they give inconsistent results. However, it is possible to reconstruct the varicose networks anatomically to restore healthy blood circulation and prevent relapses.

7
Emotional Disorders should not hide Organic Impotence

Sexual disagreement and psychological blocking explain impotence in some instances. To allot it exclusively to emotional disorders is a mistake maintained by public rumor and lack of information. After 40 years, without preventive medication, men gradually lose their virility. It follows penile arterial contraction, venous dilation, and, sometimes, local sclerosis. Organic impotence is caused by the deficiency of testicular secretion in men with an androgenic disease of andropause.

In 1972, Perlman and Kobashi studied the incidence of impotence in a series of 2,801 men [1]. These statistics show that 5 percent of *untreated* men are impotent at around forty years. This percentage then rises to 85 percent at about 80 years.

With age, erections become difficult, unstable, or absent. In some cases, hard nuclei caused by sclerosis develop in the penis and cause the deviation of erections, sometimes making any sexual intercourse impossible.

Weak Erections

Weak erections are caused by arterial insufficiency, venous escape, or nervous lesions.

Arterial Insufficiency

The arterial insufficiency of the penis is a frequent consequence of an androgenic disease of andropause.

Percentage of impotent men at various ages [1].	
Age in years	Percent of impotent men
40–49	5
50–59	11.3
60–69	35.6
70–79	59
80+	85

Table 1

Male hormone defects obstruct penile arteries; insufficient blood flow makes erection impossible. When arterial insufficiency is detected early enough, taking male hormones can restore sexual power entirely or partially.

Arteriosclerosis of the large arterial trunks causes vascular insufficiency in the lower extremities. As a result, the genitals' irrigation is compromised. The development and permeability of penile arteries depend selectively on adequate exposure to male hormones.

Venous Escape

Blood irrigates correctly in the penis, but an erection is not maintained. This is because the venous network, too broad, with a varicose tendency, lets blood contained in the penis continuously escape.

Radiographs of the cavernous bodies of the penis can show one or more venous escapes. Binding the abnormal veins and eliminating the varicose networks can treat this cause of organic impotence.

However, the venous walls consist of slackened elastic tissues and are sclerosed in the absence of male hormones. Therefore, the maintenance of an erection depends on the good hormonal impregnation of the venous network.

Nervous Lesions

Erection depends on the integrity of the nervous system. Neuronal impotence is caused by a lesion of the genital nerves or a pathology of sexual centers in the spinal cord or the brain. The impotence can result from a section of the genitals' nerves in the bladder or rectum surgery when a tumor imposes the total ablation of one of the organs. The sensitivity of the erectile tissue also depends on adequate levels of male hormones.

Curved Erection

An erection is curved when one of the walls of the penis is shorter than the other. This anomaly results from a congenital malformation or sclerosis of the cavernous bodies. A curved erection sometimes makes sexual penetration impossible.

François de La Peyronie *first* described the sclerosis of the cavernous bodies. The development in the penis of one or several hard cores, sometimes painful, causes the deviation and the deformation of the penis in erection. In addition, hormonal lack induced the progressive invasion of the erectile body by fibrous tissue in segments of the penis that are too rigid. This fibrosis develops mainly in the middle of the penis, between the two sponge-like regions of erectile tissue, which contain most of the blood in the penis during an erection. It can extend over the entire length of the penis or be localized in one or more cores.

Fibrosis begins at the periphery of the penis. Still, it can extend toward its center by blocking, each time more, the progression of blood flow through fibrosis and the arterial obstruction itself, which accompanies the degenerative process.

It is likely that arterial obstruction is initially responsible for the fibrous thickening of the cavernous envelopes. Installed fibrosis worsens the circulatory deficit, which supports fibrosis: it is the typical example of a pathological vicious circle. During a healthy erection, the penis is filled to its top and is straight and rigid.

In the event of fibrous cores, blood flow across the obstacle is poor; the penis is curved, with a rigid cord underlying two tumescent segments. In extreme cases, the penis in erection presents the form of a right angle, but all aspects are possible from five to ninety degrees, generally upward and laterally. Penetration is still possible with a penis at a small angle, but a large curve is impossible. The fibrous process worsens, and blood no longer crosses the obstacle. The top of the penis does not inflate and stays soft and cold despite good tumescence ahead of the fibrous segment. Then the roots of the cavernous bodies become fibrous, the penis is hardened, tumescence is increasingly difficult to obtain, and finally, any sexual relationship is impossible.

The clinical evolution of the disease can be slow or extend over several years. Extremely fast regressions exist; the sex act is unrealizable in two or three months, even in young men. Sometimes the induration worsens temporarily and reabsorbs entirely without drugs.

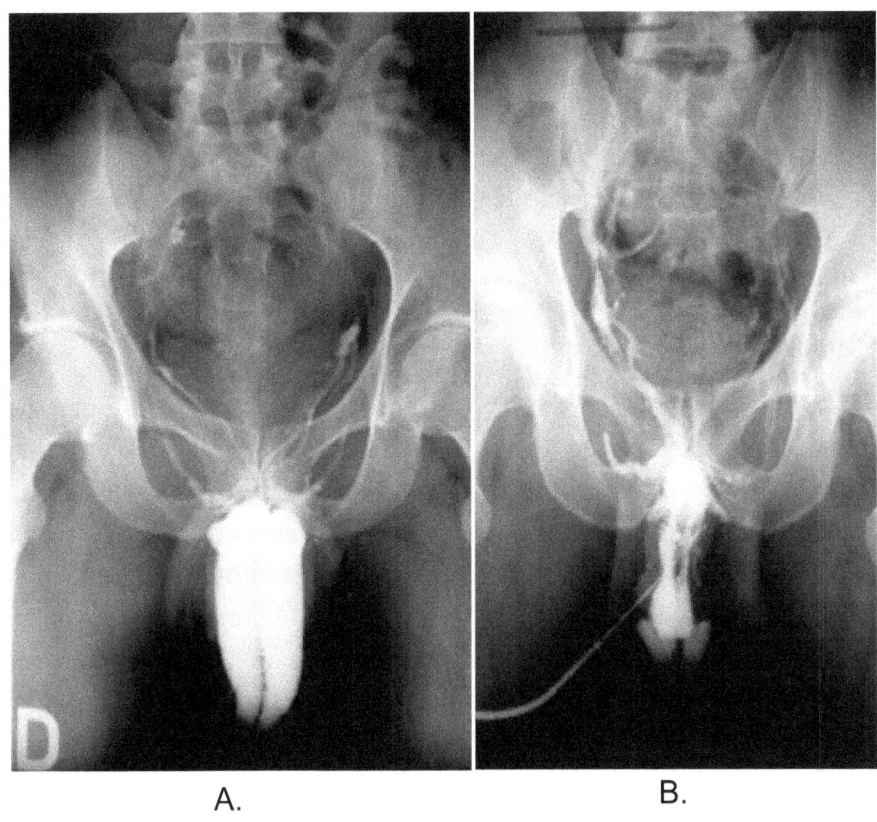

Fig. 4

A: Radiographs of healthy cavernous bodies
B: Radiographs of cavernous bodies' sclerosis

Treatment

Why do penile arteries present these phenomena of arteriosclerosis in young and older adults? First, the vascularization of the genitals is especially sensitive to hormonal influence, as is the entire genital region.

Men with cavernous body sclerosis can have disturbances in sex hormone metabolism. The balance of male hormones can control this. Taking male hormones at the beginning of the disease can make the induration disappear. When lesions have formed over several years, hormonal treatment can stabilize the condition.

The Diagnosis of Sexual Ageing

Clinical History

The history of this fifty-two-year-old man is characteristic. For a few months, nothing has gone well. He is in a gloomy mood, discouraged, and cannot concentrate. He rises tired and arrives late at his office several times in the morning, which has never happened before. He has already heard several remarks. However, he fears losing his job, which he is doing with increasing difficulty. He regularly visits the convalescent home where his parents live. He took care of them with much devotion, but these visits became increasingly challenging to make. He has two sons, one eighteen years old, the other twenty. Their friends unceasingly invade his home. The stir they cause continues to irritate him. However, six months ago, everything was fine. He was a happy man and had succeeded in his job. Now, it all seems too heavy. Yesterday, unfortunately, he had an unexplained sexual breakdown. The same mishap occurred the previous week. His wife said nothing, but he realized she had been asking herself questions. Did he take a mistress? Doesn't she like him anymore? Nothing of that sort. The breakdowns are unexplainable. He goes to the doctor to get the truth.

"I do not know how to explain," he says, embarrassedly.

"What happened?"

"I have a feeling I'm becoming impotent."

"Don't you have sex anymore? Any intercourse?"

"To tell the truth, no. I have erections, but they are increasingly rare. I have been very occupied lately, and I thought it would pass. But the situation worsens rather. I broke down sexually two consecutive times in fifteen days. I don't understand."

"Six months ago, everything was fine?"

"Yes, rather well. But while reflecting, it seems to me that I'd already felt a decrease in sexual activity one year ago, perhaps even before.

"Have you had serious diseases?"

"No."

"Did you undergo surgery, even during early childhood?"

"No, not to my recollection."

"It is most probably that your andropause is responsible for your state."

"My andropause?"

"Yes. After forty years, any man undergoes, one day or another, a fall in his sexual activity because his testicles do not secrete enough male hormones anymore. Nobody escapes it."

"Is it a kind of menopause for men?"

"It is comparable, indeed."

"Is this definitive?"

"Yes. Your sexual program started with puberty; it finishes now. Formerly, men remained in this state; fortunately, today, it is possible to correct the testicles' deficiency by taking male hormones."

"You reassure me. What is necessary to do?"

"A blood test will determine your hormone levels. Then, I will prescribe you a treatment, considering the results."

After being examined and receiving the analysis request, Bob goes to the laboratory the following day. He states, "I am hurrying to know the results a few days later."

"They are not brilliant. I suspected it. Your testosterone level is low: 400 ng/mL. It is the average rate for an eighty-year-old man; some even have a higher rate. I will prescribe you hormones for three months, and then we will control the results."

Three months later.

The doctor asks, "What is the news?"

"Everything is fine. I recovered all my sexual capacities. My wife is delighted. Even my general state has improved. I'm in good shape. I enjoy working, and I am busy with projects. I have the feeling that nothing can stop me anymore."

"Perfect. We will continue the same treatment with weaker amounts for one year."

"Is it necessary to continue to take hormones? I thought that the treatment was finished."

"It has only begun. The secretion of your testicles will remain insufficient throughout your life. It is necessary to replace what they no longer produce. If you stop the treatment, everything will start again."

"I do not want that."

"Here are your prescriptions. We will see each other again for annual control."

While following his treatment regularly, he did not have problems anymore. His history is that of a million men with andropause. How many follow the procedure? The number is ridiculous — a few hundred in France and a few thousand worldwide. Many men consult too late when their genitals have completely deteriorated. The lack of hormones is added to mechanical problems of erections, blocked arteries, or dilated veins, sometimes all three.

LEVELS OF SEX HORMONE

The Normal Testosterone Level in Blood

Whatever one's age, the low testosterone metabolism causes a lack of libido, passivity, general tiredness, and unexplained depression. Let us first define the word "normal." The dictionary says, "What is applied to the greatest number." In this case, healthy would be the average. But nothing is more singular than the individual structure. Each man presents a hormonal configuration. Therefore, he does not have to be treated according to the standard of the whole population.

However, to get some fixed ideas, the plasmatic testosterone average level is as follows:

Age in years	Nanograms/100 mL
Between 20 and 30	1000 to 700
Between 30 and 60	700 to 600
Between 60 and 80	440 to 400

Table 2

Laboratories often locate the testosterone level on a scale that goes from three hundred to nine hundred nanograms per 100 milliliters of plasma. It is an uninterpretable statistical concept because all men are located on this scale. They have a rate of nine hundred at twenty years and three hundred at one hundred.

A testosterone rate lower than three hundred nanograms per one hundred milliliters of plasma is compatible with hypogonadism.

The Level of Dihydrotestosterone

The production of dihydrotestosterone reflects the sexual organs' activity. A level of 90 nanograms per 100 milliliters of plasma indicates good activity. Twenty-five nanograms per hundred milliliters of plasma represent weak sexual activity.

Here, laboratories often set "normal" levels at 25 nanograms per 100 milliliters of plasma. All men are on this scale: ninety at twenty to twenty-five at one hundred years.

The Free Testosterone Level

With age, testosterone is released less from its carrying proteins. Therefore, the ideal percentage of free testosterone is 2 percent at 20 years.
Suppose one considers the normal range from 20 to 30 years. In that case, the quantity of free testosterone in plasma ranges between 140 and 200 picograms per milliliter (a picogram is a thousandth of a billionth of a gram), an unceasingly renewed, modest amount. The action of testosterone depends on its free molecules, which enter cells and initiate a reaction.

The Daily Production of Testosterone

The testicles must produce from seven to ten milligrams of testosterone daily, accounting for seven to ten million nanograms. When this production decreases, the blood/testosterone rate drops, and the sex hormone profile is disturbed. That means that a biochemical imbalance is underway.

The proportioning of daily testosterone production is not yet achievable in current practice. But with a simple blood test and the determination of various levels of male hormones, it is possible to do a good job. The interpretation of hormonal proportioning is sensitive and must be made by a doctor aware of hormone therapy and knowledgeable about the pathology of the genitals. The advice of the family doctor can also be helpful.

The interpretation of hormonal results is based solely on analyses performed by specialized laboratories and rigorous analytical methods.

The Level of Female Hormones

The testicle produces a female hormone, estradiol. In peripheral blood, estradiol reaches a concentration of 20 picograms per milliliter of plasma (determined by radioimmunoassay).

An estradiol level of eighty picograms per milliliter of plasma is compatible with a total lack of sexual instincts.

To prevent the androgenic disease of andropause, check your sex hormones and the appearance of symptoms; if you are over forty, check your hormones once a year.

Special Examinations

When a mechanical disorder of erections exists, one has several examinations to specify the diagnosis. They are a little curious but inoffensive and initially record night erections. This examination detects the swelling of the penis during sleep. It is practiced to determine the origin of impotence, whether psychic or organic. It is enough to listen well to the impotent man for knowledge, and this examination will not be necessary.

During specific periods of sleep, the penis inflates. Therefore, if it is pleasant to wake following a strong erection, one usually does not wake up at night.

The lack of swelling of the penis during the night means that the impotence is organic. The opposite situation does not allow a definitive conclusion. The night swelling of the penis does not mean potency for two reasons: first, if the penis inflates, it is not necessarily rigid. Then an erection can be paradoxical. It is the erection caused by bladder distension. Well known in the morning, it results from compression of the penis veins by a full bladder.

Prostate diseases are frequent in a man with the androgenic disease of andropause. He empties his bladder badly and is generally impotent. He often rises at night to urinate, and the distension of his bladder can cause several passive night erections.

When prostatism is the consequence of sexual ageing, the man who presents a passive erection at night is often unable to obtain an active erection. For him, the blood contribution is insufficient to ensure an erection if there is no venous compression (by the full bladder), slowing down the venous return. This paradox commonly results in the expression, "I have an erection when I should not have one. But unfortunately, I do not have any when I should have."

To evaluate the insufficiency of the irrigation of the penis and locate the level of the arterial obstruction, one uses the Doppler effect (name of its inventor) process to determine the speed of a vehicle. The radar sends an ultrasound wave toward the car, which is reflected back to the radar receiver. The frequency variation between the emitted and reflected waves depends on the vehicle's speed.

The Doppler effect applied to the arterial network and the arteries of the penis provides invaluable information on the propagation velocity of the blood wave. The transmitter and receiver of blood waves are in a pencil-sized probe that is applied to the studied artery. The sensor is connected to an electronic unit that enables the graphical and audio representation of blood flow speed.

The radiological study of the cavernous bodies is obtained by injecting a contrast liquid directly into the penis. This puncture is no more painful than that necessary to take a blood sample. The solution is injected drop by drop.

Each case of impotence is evaluated according to the state of the arterial and venous networks; an erection is helpful if blood flow is normal and venous outflow is unimpeded.

Treatment

Male hormones treat the cause of impotence since they are missing in men with the androgenic disease of andropause. When the therapy is undertaken at the beginning of the disease, it is possible to restore blood circulation in the penis and avoid impotence. Unfortunately, many men are unaware of this cause and gradually become impotent. After several years of hormonal lack, it can be impossible to reconstitute a sufficient vascularization to maintain an erection through hormonal treatment, which may prevent the progression of impotence and is always necessary.

Ejaculation Disorders

The seminal vesicles secrete most parts of the spermatic fluid. Ejaculation occurs when the genital ways are inflated by sperm, and the nerve centers are stimulated. This natural phenomenon occurs in young men two or three times per week.

When there is no sexual activity (for example, for religious reasons in certain priests), genital ways are filled gradually, and ejaculation occurs automatically, generally at night during erotic dreams. So it is often the case in a teenager who does not masturbate and finds his stained sheets from wet dreams when he awakes.

A young priest consults the doctor because his nocturnal emissions make him feel guilty due to his religion. But nature is nature, and there is nothing abnormal. Formerly, some monks wanted to be castrated to avoid temptation. However, the Christian Church prohibited this solution, as the Council of Nicaea (325 AD) held that overcoming temptation in this way had no merit.

When the contraction of the genital ways is not accompanied by ejaculation, the pressure created sometimes causes intense pain. This phenomenon often occurs in teenagers who do not have a sexual partner and do not masturbate. Masturbation is not shameful; certain monks affirm that it is not reprehensible if the intention is pure.

Disorders of Ejaculation, Real Causes, and Treatment

Disorders of ejaculation are varied and more frequent than generally thought.

The androgenic disease of andropause causes the regression of all genital functions. Therefore, ejaculation is less frequent and can become painful, early, or delayed. In addition, ejaculation without a firm erection is a sign of sexual decrepitude.

The production of sperm reduces at the time of andropause. It frequently happens that ejaculation reduces to a drop; sometimes, it becomes impossible: the creation of sperm has stopped. It explains, among other things, the reduction in the frequency of sexual intercourse.

Carl Pearlman and Luis Kobashi studied the frequency of sexual intercourse in 2,801 men of all ages [1].

Ages in years	Percentage of men who have sexual intercourse once per week or more
20	88
40	80
50	68
60	50
70	25
80	10

Table 3

As one would expect, the frequency of sexual activity varies directly according to age, young people being the most active. The reduction in sexual activity parallels the fall of male hormone secretions.

Painful ejaculation is a sign of irritation of the genital ways caused by the senile involution of the genitals. The cause can be mechanical, infectious, or congestive.

Premature Ejaculation

Ejaculation is a nervous reflex that answers the physical excitation of the genitals or an erotogenic stimulation of the cerebral sexual centers. One can ejaculate thanks to masturbation without having an intense orgasm. On the other hand, ejaculation can occur under the effect of an uncontrolled emotion, with an orgasm without genital physical stimulation. When everything concurs, there is no problem.

When premature ejaculation occurs only once, it is accidental. However, when the phenomenon repeats, it becomes worrying.

Premature ejaculation of organic origin generally occurs in all circumstances of the sexual act without being able to allot its cause to fear or excessive psychic stimulation.

Any excessive stimulation at a point of the reflex arc accelerates the nervous reaction and causes premature ejaculation. It was believed that premature ejaculation was always psychological because the organic causes were ignored. However, it is known today that anomalies caused by sexual ageing are frequent. They irritate the nervous reflex in various places: the foreskin, the ejaculatory ducts, and the ejaculation glands.

Sex hormones directly influence the skin of the penis. Therefore, the foreskin becomes delicate, fragile, and sensitive when there is a lack of male hormones. Its sensitivity causes premature ejaculation, which a good hormonal impregnation will restore.

A fragile foreskin is easily infected by viruses (herpes), mycoses, and germs. The infection is sometimes such that circumcision is necessary.

Sometimes a rigid ring forms, making it impossible to uncover the glans. This ring of sclerosis can result from a hormonal deficiency.

Infection of the prostate, ejaculatory ducts, and seminal vesicles disturbs ejaculation and must be eliminated with antibiotics and local treatment.

Premature ejaculation for medical reasons can benefit from the installation of penile implants. The speed of ejaculation does not change in each case, but sexual activity becomes possible. This case is rare.

I operated many years ago on a thirty-year-old man who was a premature ejaculator. He was on the edge of suicide despite many psychiatric treatments. He had never had a healthy sexual activity before. After his implant surgery, ejaculation became standardized. He married and has since lived in total harmony. He became the father of two little boys.

Delayed Ejaculation

The purpose of certain erotic games is to delay, for a long time, the moment of ejaculation. In other, less happy circumstances, ejaculation is hindered by the inexperience or the indifference of two partners, whatever the age. Sexual ageing reduces sperm secretion. Ejaculated volume decreases gradually with time. In extreme cases, ejaculation becomes impossible. When a man ejaculates little after a very long time, when the orgasm decreases or disappears, it is necessary to think about sexual ageing, even in young men. Hormonal disorders can be responsible for this sexual regression and must be corrected.

The genital-urinary tract in regression is easily. As a result, the lack of sexual desire develops insidiously. A defect in male hormones and an excess of female hormones can be responsible for this sexual regression.

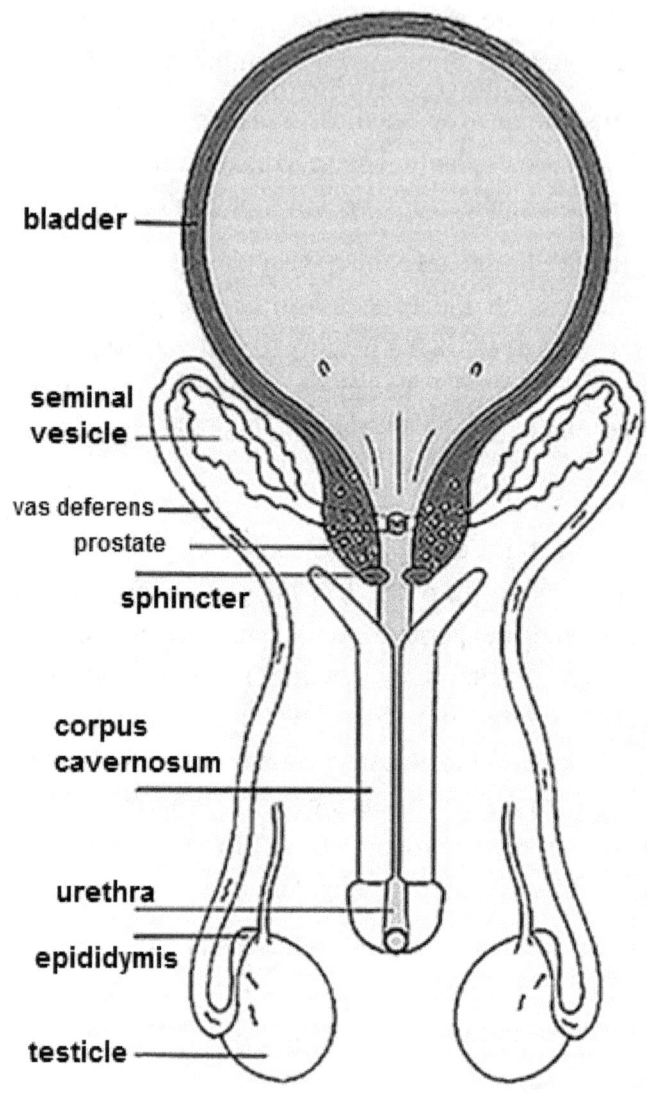

Fig. 5

Anatomy of the male genital apparatus

9

Prostate Problems

The Prostate is not only a Gland

There is great confusion in the literature about the definition of this organ. The prostate is not a gland, contrary to the summary definitions of dictionaries and some medical books. What do dictionaries say? "Prostate: also called prostate gland, is a gland in male mammals that surrounds the neck of the bladder and urethra and secretes a liquid constituent of the semen" (*Collins English Dictionary*).

The prostate is a compound tubuloalveolar exocrine gland of the male reproductive system in most mammals. It differs considerably among species anatomically, chemically, and physiologically. The function of the prostate is to secrete a slightly alkaline fluid, milky or white in appearance" (*Wikipedia*). "Prostate: an organ near the penis in male mammals that produces a liquid that mixes with and carries sperm" (Cambridge Advanced Learner's Dictionary & Thesaurus).

What does the treaty of the anatomy of H. Rouvière say? "The prostate is a glandular structure which surrounds in man the initial part of the urethra" [1].

Those definitions lack precision. They mention only the glandular structure of the prostate. The idea commonly follows that the prostate is a gland whose function is exclusively sexual. That is inaccurate.

Diagrams and drawings in books representing the prostate are generally approximate and muddle understanding. Furthermore, the seminal vesicles secrete most of the spermatic fluid.

The Prostate is a muscular structure that contains glands

Chèvremont M. describes the prostate precisely in *Notions of Cytology and Histology*, published in 1956 by Desoer editions: "The prostate is a muscular structure that contains glands more or less developed according to individuals. This structure surrounds the first portion of the urethra" [2].

The prostate muscular structure opens large during urination at the same time as the bladder neck opening (which constitutes the narrowest bladder portion made of muscle fibers), which opens the bladder exit during urination (figure 8, page 84).

In the upper part of the prostatic structure, muscular elements prevail over glandular elements. It is in continuity with the bladder neck musculature. The role of this muscular structure is to take part in the opening of the posterior urethra during urination. The bladder neck and prostate are sensitive to sex hormones. Therefore, they are organs under hormonal influence.

Urination is closely related to the integrity of the prostate's muscular structure. Therefore, excess fibrosis or muscular anomalies can explain urination difficulties in men who are not carriers of benign or malignant tumors of the glandular elements.

Men presenting fibrosis or muscular prostate structure anomalies are often young. Disorders of urination from which they suffer are qualified in the medical literature as "prostatism without prostate," which does not make sense (even a male baby has a prostate). Those disorders are shown as mental health disorders, and those men live physical and psychological martyrdom. This situation is even more deplorable, as this condition is treatable.

Hormonal imbalance leads to the development of rigid conjunctive tissue or to uncontrolled growth of the vesical neck muscle fibers.

Sometimes, the whole prostatic musculature is involved. The opening mechanism of the bladder outlet is blocked, leading to urinary disorders, while the prostate volume is not increased.

Total or partial prostate atrophy is a consequence of all deficiencies in male hormones. I described this syndrome in 1980 in the *Bulletins and Memoirs of the Société de Médecine de Paris,* an article titled "Fibrous prostate associated with an excess of female hormone." [3]. This illustrated publication left no doubt about the reality of this new pathology.

In 1971, I first described unknown pathologies in children. At that time, some children presented giant ureters whose cause was unknown. It was the primary megaureter without an apparent reason. The urine did not flow well into the bladder. The old medical dogma asserted that these were nerve malformations. And that consequently, it was useless to operate on these children, which led them irremediably to artificial kidneys and death. My study has shown that the giant dilated ureter was not due to nervous malformations but to abnormalities of the ureter's musculature, which were replaced by fibrous tissue (a kind of scar tissue). After removing the diseased part, these ureters returned to normal function, and the children were saved [4-5]. Since then, surgery has become a practice. This study began in 1962 and required 9 years of work in the laboratory of pathological anatomy at the University of Brussels, directed at the time by Professor Dustin, one of my supervisors of aggregation in urologic sciences. I performed 50,000 histological sections of normal and pathological ureters. From which seven thousand were colored with three colors (trichromatic of Masson) [4]. This work was partly published in the Medico-surgical Paris Encyclopedia [5]. By continuing my training as a urologist during this period, I noted many inconsistencies relating to pathologies of sexual and urinary organs.

My pathology studies described the genital and urinary structures surrounding the bladder exit: the bladder neck and the prostate. Discoveries were immediate. ***Histological cuts confirmed that the prostate was a muscular structure*** [2]. And pathological tissues in prostatism cases showed prostate musculature anomalies [3-4]. Thus, I understood that the expression "prostatism without prostate" sometimes used in medicine did not correspond to reality.

Hormonal analyses have existed, thanks to radioimmunology, since 1974. I showed that the insufficiency in male hormones or an excess of female hormones was the cause of many cases of prostate fibrosis [3]. It is necessary to know this pathology to understand sexual ageing. Unfortunately, it is still largely ignored, decades after I first described it to several medical societies.

Atrophy of the prostate is a mechanical and functional obstacle responsible for hypertension upstream in the urinary tract, destroying the kidneys [4]. However, the prostate structure is generally ignored because medical books and dictionaries poorly define it. It is consequently impossible to treat pathologies of an organ whose structure is not understood.

Prostate Atrophy

Reduction in the secretion of male hormones and hormone imbalance always causes structural modifications in the prostate, producing urination disorders.

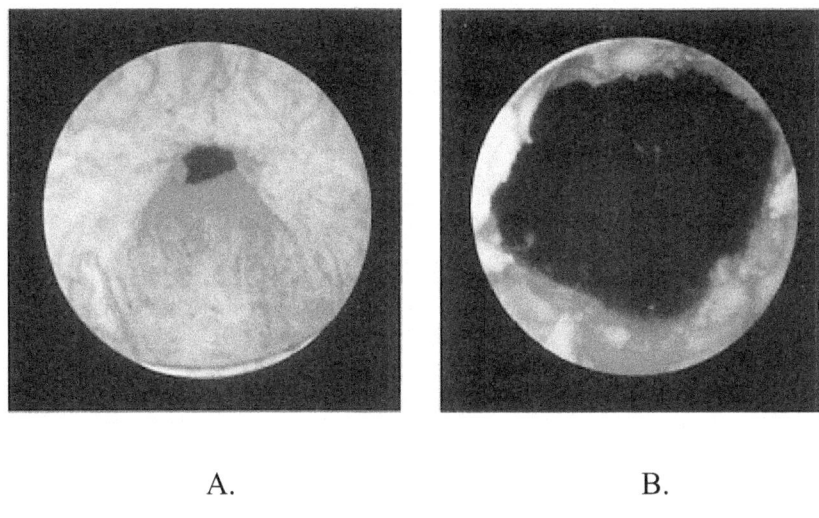

A.   B.

Fig. 6

A. The endoscopic aspect of an atrophied prostate. The duct is narrow and encircled by rigid fibrous tissue (five millimeters). The redness of walls characterizes congestive vascularization.

B. The endoscopic aspect of the prostate after removal of diseased tissue. The diameter of the prostatic duct is five centimeters. Previously, the width was five millimeters (A).

Prostate Atrophy Caused by Dangerous Drugs

The best example is baldness, for which 5α-reductase inhibitors are prescribed to reduce dihydrotestosterone formation in hair follicles, aiming to slow hair loss. Unfortunately, by doing this, inhibitors of 5α-reductase also penetrate the prostate structures—which depend on dihydrotestosterone—causing their atrophy with disastrous consequences. In addition, 5α-reductase inhibitors produce effects similar to those of androgenic disease.

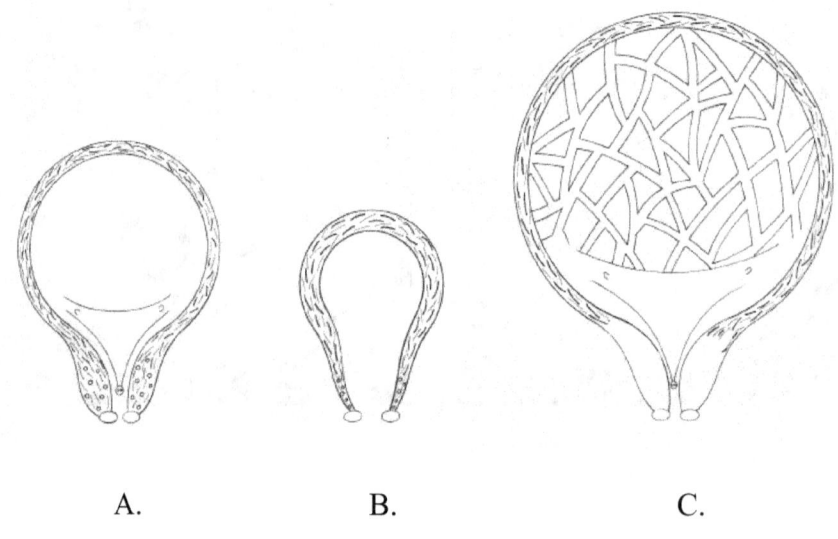

A.   B.   C.

Fig. 7

Diagram of the prostate's atrophy (C)

Fig. A. The bladder musculature is anchored to the vesical neck in continuity with the prostate's muscular structure.

Fig. B. When the bladder contracts during urination, the muscular structure of the healthy prostate opens and does not offer any resistance to urine flow.

Fig. C. To lack male hormones, the atrophied prostate comprises fibrous and rigid tissue (the tissue of scars). When the bladder contracts, the posterior urethra opens badly (Figures 8-9, page 83). Muscle fibers of the bladder hypertrophy initially. Then the vesical muscle distends gradually until becoming a vast, flaccid bladder unable to be emptied.

Serial radiographs taken during urination show the funnel opening of the prostatic urethra.

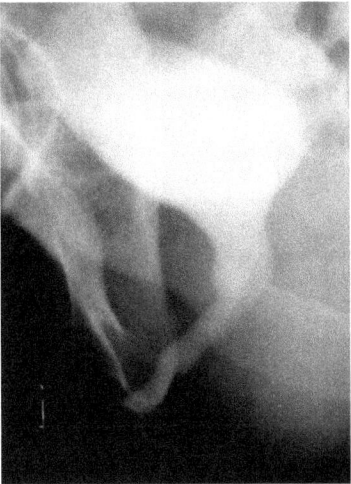

Fig. 8

A radiograph taken during urination shows the wide opening (1.5 centimeters) of the prostatic urethra.

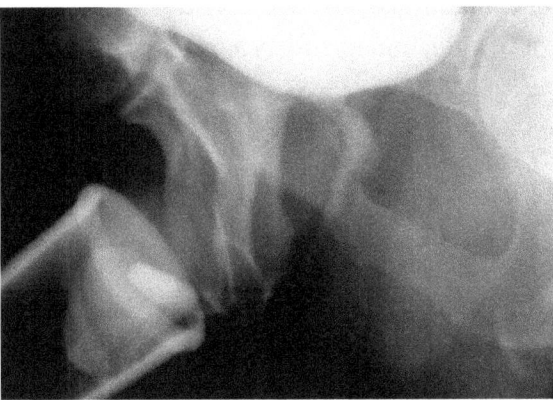

Fig. 9

A radiograph taken during urination shows a narrowing of the prostatic urethra (three millimeters) resulting from sclerosis of the prostate musculature.

Prostate Adenoma

Adenoma of the prostate is a benign tumor caused by a disordered state of the sex hormone chain. My clinical experience, renewed many times, shows that the adjustment of various sex hormones stabilizes and makes urinary symptoms disappear for many years, thus delaying surgery. The therapy of male hormone disorders requires a detailed analysis of androgen metabolism. Prostatic adenoma typically develops after age 60. Inhibitors of the 5α-reductase are often used to treat prostate adenoma, though the reader has seen that those inhibitors produce atrophy of the prostate musculature and sexual problems.

According to a US Food and Drug Administration warning, 5 million men received 5α-reductase inhibitors between 2002 and 2009. Three million of them were between the ages of fifty and seventy-nine. Taking finasteride (Proscar®, Propecia®) or Dutasteride (Advocart®, Jalyn®) to "treat" adenoma can cause more severe prostate cancer (Safety Announcement: 06-09-2011) [6]. This warning from the Food and Drug Administration supported what I affirmed decades earlier: a well-proportioned androgen treatment (and not its suppression) can stabilize the rostate adenomap and avoid surgery.

Prostate Cancer

Control of the Hormonal Balance

Prostate glands can become cancerous. Since 1974, I have been surprised by the scarcity of prostate cancer in men taking well-proportioned male hormones. The few rare cancer cases observed under precise and well-dosed androgen therapy did not present any difficulty. A suitable treatment cured them after *having profited from an early diagnosis*. On the other hand, I saw evolutionary prostate cancers in many men who did not follow any treatment with male hormones.

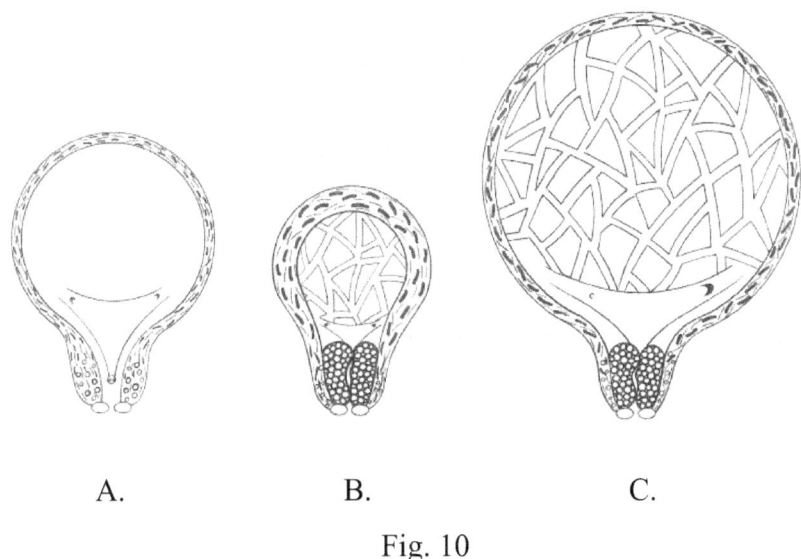

A. B. C.

Fig. 10

Diagram of the compression of the prostate's structure by an adenoma

Fig. A. The prostate is not only a gland. The prostate is a muscular structure with more or less developed glands surrounding the portion of the urethra located between the bladder neck and the sphincter. The muscular structure prevails over the glandular elements in the upper part of the prostate musculature. It is in continuity with the bladder neck musculature.

Fig. B. The hypertrophy of glands can cause the formation of a benign or malignant tumor, blocking the posterior urethra and compressing the prostate musculature. The bladder initially compensates for this difficulty by hypertrophying its musculature. The bladder's capacity is reduced, leading to frequent urination.

Fig. C. With time, the bladder muscle weakens. As a result, the large, flaccid bladder is unable to empty. Therefore, the transition from a hypertrophic state to a flaccid bladder is faster or slower, depending on the importance of the obstacle.

A significant obstruction of the urethra can quickly lead to a large, flaccid bladder. Sometimes several years are necessary to transform a hypertonic bladder into a flaccid one.

These clinical observations must be considered alongside interesting scientific studies conducted in recent years and published in 1996 by the James Buchanan Brady Urological Institute and the Johns Hopkins University School of Medicine, Baltimore, Maryland, on telomeres[*] and telomerase enzyme activity in the cells of prostates and seminal vesicles of castrated rats [7].

The authors reported increased telomerase activity[†] in seminal vesicle and prostate cells from castrated rats.

On the contrary, the administration of androgens to these same castrated rats caused a reduction in the activity of telomerase in the cells of the seminal vesicles.

The mechanism is probably the same as the one in man. Administration of androgens most probably decreases the risk of developing prostate cancer. In other words:

1. The suppression of male hormones causes an increase in the activity of healthy prostate cells toward anarchy.

2. The administration of well-proportioned male hormones for men deprived of them should prevent healthy prostate cells from developing in anarchy with an extremely high probability.

---

[*] A telomere is an area constituting the end of a chromosome. Each time a chromosome is duplicated during replication, telomeres are shortened. The telomeres become too short and fail to protect the cell, leading to its death.

[†] Telomerase is an enzyme that allows telomeres to be reconstituted, thereby protecting the cell from death.

It is necessary to undertake new clinical studies without delay to confirm that.

Pathological studies practiced during autopsies showed that the malignant transformations of the prostate (anomalies of the structure of cells) were frequent after age fifty. Cancer incidence varies from less than 30 percent at fifty to 100 percent beyond age ninety [8-9]. These observations show that tumors increase in number with age but can escape detection for years. Furthermore, these occult tumors are well-differentiated and homogeneous* [10]; they are small and unperceived. They have a slow evolution. As a result, many older men die unaware that they carry small prostate cancers.

One cannot prevent oneself from comparing the increase in the frequency of prostate cancer after age fifty with the progressive lowering of the secretion of male hormones. But unfortunately, the two phenomena follow opposite curves and progress with age.

Unknown a few years ago, diagnostic tests for prostate cancer are available today. The association of examinations by a scanner† or nuclear magnetic resonance‡, echography, prostate biopsy guided by

---

* The differentiated cancer cells do not present the typical anarchistic histological characteristics of invading cancer cells.
Histology: The science that treats the structure of tissues and cells constituting living beings.

† Scanner: apparatus of radio diagnosis made up of a system of tomography and a computer which reconstitutes the data on a screen. Synonym: Tomodensitometry.
Tomography: a radiological process of exploration having the goal to obtain radiography of a thin layer of the body to a desired depth

‡ Nuclear magnetic resonance (N.M.R.) is a radiological process that uses the magnetic properties of tissues to highlight their structures. The images reconstituted by the computer are of extraordinary precision.

echography, and knowledge of specific tumor markers in blood already makes it possible to detect cancers of 5 millimeters.

The prostate cancer not detected by these powerful means of diagnosis is inevitably microscopic. Let us imagine that it consists of some cells in an older man that contain male hormone receptors (an essential condition for activation). This man still makes a modest quantity of male hormones, and cells bathe literally in a "testosterone bath." Indeed, a man with an androgenic andropause disease does not provide more than three milligrams of testosterone per day (the average production is seven milligrams per day). Nevertheless, he puts 3 billion picograms of testosterone into circulation daily, produced by his body. It would be sufficient to activate some cancer cells. Treatment of the androgenic disease of andropause with well-proportioned and well-adapted androgens (mesterolone) is safe. There is no risk in enabling an infraclinical prostate cancer with therapeutic quantities, that is, by restoring normal levels of male hormones in the blood.

A lack of male hormones causes prostate atrophy and, consequently, the weakness of its structure. Studies of small prostate cancers show that the atrophied and compressed zones, apart from the nodules of benign hypertrophy, are the privileged place for cancer [11]. Therefore, prostate atrophy and prostate cancer should not be considered as isolated entities. These pathologies must be placed in their context: a degenerated body no longer defended, as it undergoes the degenerative phenomena of androgenic disease of andropause, including immune deficiency*.

The correction of hormonal imbalance can constitute a method of prostate cancer prevention. There are two reasons, one epidemiologic and the other histological.

---

* Testosterone is an immune regulator, a property that makes an organism refractory to certain pathogens.

The correction of hormonal imbalance can constitute a method of prostate cancer prevention. There are two reasons, one epidemiologic and the other histological.

• In 1988, a study relating to a population of 6,860 men followed for nearly fourteen years, the Japan-Hawaii Cancer Study [12], shows that *the imbalance and the deficit of sex hormones are significant*. Ninety-eight men with advanced prostate cancer in a group were compared to men of the same age having a healthy prostate.

• At the beginning of the destructive processes, the prostate cells are still relatively well differentiated. In tissue culture, prostate cells become more regular in the presence of testosterone [13].

These two case studies probably explain the absence of invading prostatic cancer in men following a well-proportioned androgen therapy for many years. In addition, this treatment prevents the degeneration of the prostate as an organ.

Three Great Errors to Be Avoided Concerning Prostate Cancer

• Error 1: To believe that PSA is a specific marker of prostate cancer.

The PSA is a marker of cell activity. Its level in the blood ranges from 1 to 4 nanograms per milliliter. An infection of the prostate can cause a rise in PSA levels. Prostate adenoma can also raise this level. On the contrary, invasive prostate cancer exists that does not secrete PSA

Since its appearance on the market, the PSA (prostate-specific antigen) has been used as a specific marker of prostate cancer. PSA was then used to determine the effectiveness of various treatments.

Doctors, in general, put in decades before realizing that the PSA level does not make it possible to distinguish aggressive prostate cancer from well-tolerated prostate cancer, which led to abusive diagnoses and unnecessarily aggressive treatments.

<u>In the United States, insurers do not cover the detection of the PSA level for the preventive diagnosis of prostate cancer.</u>

• **Error 2: To believe that testosterone causes the cancerous transformation of prostate cells by confusing the action of this male hormone on various "states" of the prostate cells.**

There are 10 degrees of prostate cell transformation, from the most benign to the most malignant. These transformations are known as <u>Gleason</u>'s grades.

The first five grades correspond to transformations that can regress toward the typical structure <u>under the influence of male hormones</u> [13]—in other words, to regress from grade five toward grade four toward the inoffensive degree one. The first six grades of the transformation can correspond to a rise in PSA levels, which can decrease under the influence of <u>well-proportioned male hormones.</u>

Male hormones can stimulate aggressive grades of cellular transformation, from 7 to 10, in a culture of tissues and, consequently, clinically. If the level of PSA rises under hormone androgens, the treatment is unnecessary or contraindicated. That can constitute an element for the early diagnosis of invasive prostate cancer.

• **Error 3: To ignore the in vivo biological balance between testosterone and dihydrotestosterone**

•

Is It Still Necessary to Remove Male Hormones from Patients with Prostate Cancer?

The problem of prostate cancer is very particular. First, the cause of prostate cancer is not known. Considering the therapeutic problem with hindsight is advisable, especially given our vast ignorance. The treatment of prostate cancer is complex and would require writing a whole book.

Is cancer localized? Is it invading the pelvis? Is it generalized? Many questions will be answered based on the singularity of the concerned person and the uniqueness of his cancer cells.

One of the therapeutic approaches consists of neutralizing the action of male hormones by various means that cause sexual impotence:

• administration of female hormones.

• administration of hormones that block the action of testosterone (acetate of cyproterone).

• partial suppression of androgen secretion by the organism, practicing the ablation of testicular tissues (the testicles' contents are removed)—in this case, the production of androgens by the suprarenal glands persists.

• total suppression of androgen secretion by the organism, practicing a chemical castration. The androgens from the testicles and suprarenal glands are then blocked.

Treatment with female hormones (estrogen) was in vogue until 1967. This year, a famous study of the veterans' hospitals in the United States concluded, "Although the treatment with estrogens has an initial beneficial effect among certain patients, this effect is more than compensated for by an increase in consecutive mortality from cardiovascular complications" [14].

Physical or chemical castration, antiandrogens, and complete inhibition of male hormone secretion were used [15]. Total suppression of male hormones can stabilize generalized cancers to some extent (none have ever been cured). But does not the tree hide the forest? Under such conditions, all the structures of the body also degenerate.

It is still necessary to consider the astonishing clinical results of generalized prostate cancers treated with male hormones [16-17]. All the other therapeutic measures having failed, these treatments were undertaken in cases of disseminated disease and sometimes produced spectacularly favorable results, probably because of the revitalization of the body and its defenses. Unfortunately, these exceptional cases do nothing but delay the fatal date.

In 2001, researchers at the University of Western Australia in Perth showed that the suppression of male hormones by chemical castration among patients with prostate cancer causes β-amyloid protein deposits in the brain. One finds these deposits in Alzheimer's disease (chapter 29 [10]) One will realize, in a few years, that patients with prostate cancer "died cured" at the end of the twentieth century and the beginning of the twenty-first century, thanks to the complete suppression of their male hormones, as was the case for the use of female hormones before 1967.

Symptoms of Prostatism

The urinary stream becomes weak. Many men do not worry and do not find it abnormal to not urinate as well at age sixty as they did at age twenty. They ignore their prostate's ageing. Gradually, the urinary stream becomes threadlike, and urination may become a drip. Finally, the bladder no longer empties, and it is no longer possible to pass a single urine drop.

Transfer to the hospital with a bladder containing several liters is always dramatic until the moment when a saving probe comes to deflate the bladder. Then the sick prostate will be removed.

Getting up at night to urinate is regarded as self-explanatory with age. This observation is part of the collective memory, and an older man is often unaware of its importance. At first, he urinates once during the night. Months and years pass. He gets up then twice or three times. Certain men wait to urinate ten times per night to be alarmed because they can no longer sleep and are very tired. Pain while urinating and bloody urine are more spectacular and encourage the man with an androgenic disease of andropause to consult his doctor as soon as possible. These troubles can result from a lack of prevention or treatment with male hormones. Therefore, it is necessary to be conscious and make an early diagnosis of androgenic disease of andropause. In the absence of symptoms, it is helpful, after age forty, to regularly have blood tests to detect biological decline at its earliest stages. The sick prostate diagnosis is made by a digital rectal exam, an examination of prostate secretions under the microscope, recording urinated volume according to time, prostate echography, radiography while urinating (figures 8,9; page 84), and determination in the blood of a specific protein secreted by prostate glands, the PSA*.

The codependence of hormones and prostate cancer is more difficult to detect. People with cancerous illnesses generally have "normal" levels (for their age) or reduced levels of male hormones. The hormonal study of prostate cancer patients should be more advanced, as it is almost inevitable that prostate cancer generally develops around age seventy, when the hormonal upheavals are considerable. Therefore, control of

---

* The level of PSA (prostatic-specific antigen) in blood is normally between two and a half and four nanograms per milliliter of plasma. Higher levels indicate an abnormal activity of the prostate glands.

hormonal metabolism should be a priority of medical research and public health [18-19].

Endoscopic Treatments

Infection settles in when a prostatic obstacle causes poor bladder draining. To solve a chronic infectious problem, it is sometimes necessary to eliminate the prostatic obstruction. Endoscopic surgery allows the removal of pathologic tissue with millimeter-level precision.

The sphincter (annular musculature surrounding a natural opening, closing it while contracting) extends by one centimeter. The fear of incontinence, propagated by public rumors, is unjustified if one studies the field of endoscopy. Final postoperative incontinence results from a surgical defect, the sphincter having been injured. The patient who is continent before surgery must be continent afterward.

It is impossible to understand general ageing and its diseases without first understanding genital and urinary ageing.

That's half a century that I have been repeating it. Nevertheless, I do not weary myself and will continue to repeat it until it is no longer necessary.

Part III

Diseases of Ageing

One dies in detail, my dear friend;
may you enjoy a better
health than mine.

VOLTAIRE

Correspondence,
November 17, 1764

10

Diabetes and Androgenic disease of andropause: The Sugar Mechanism

In 2011, there were 347 million diabetic people with diabetes globally [1]. The World Health Organization (WHO) predicts that, in 2030, diabetes will be the seventh-leading cause of death worldwide [2].

Key Facts

The World Health Organization (WHO) notes the following diabetes facts:

- The number of people with diabetes rose from 108 million in 1980 to 422 million in 2014.
- The global prevalence of diabetes among adults over eighteen rose from 4.7 percent in 1980 to 8.5 percent in 2014.
- Diabetes prevalence has been growing more rapidly in middle and low-income countries.
- Diabetes is a significant cause of blindness, kidney failure, heart attacks, stroke, and lower limb amputation.
- In 2016, an estimated 1.6 million deaths were directly caused by diabetes. Another 2.2 million deaths were attributable to high blood glucose in 2012.
- Almost half of all deaths due to high blood glucose occur before the age of seventy years; the WHO estimates that diabetes was the seventh-leading cause of death in 2016.
- A healthy diet, regular physical activity, maintaining an average body weight, and avoiding tobacco use are ways to prevent or delay the onset of type 2 diabetes.

- Diabetes can be treated, and its consequences can be avoided or delayed with diet, physical activity, medication, and regular screening and treatment for complications.

According to the WHO, diabetes will be the seventh-leading cause of death in 2030 [2].

The Sugar Mechanism

The human body needs energy to function. The food contains three great sources of energy—sugars, fats, and proteins. The energy (fuel) supplied immediately is stored in sugars and fats. Glucose (sugar) is used instantaneously by the organism's cells. Proteins play a specific role, as we will see later.

Billions of glucose molecules cross the cells of the organism at every moment. They are an energy source that is immediately usable by each cell. Some sugars are stored in the liver and muscles as a reserve for use during strenuous efforts or periods of fasting. According to their composition, assimilation of sugars occurs immediately or slowly. "Fast" sugars (e.g., the sugar in honey and extremely concentrated granulated sugar) are quickly digested by the intestines, causing an immediate rise in blood sugar levels, and are used by the organism immediately. "Slow" sugars (e.g., the starch in bread, pasta, and potatoes) are composed of subunits of glucose released gradually during digestion in the intestine. As a result, they slowly raise_blood sugar levels over an extended period.

Fats contain fatty acids; fats include butter, margarine, and oils, such as sunflower, groundnut, and olive oil.

Fatty acids give fats their essential characteristics. They are soluble in fat solvents (e.g., acetone, ether, benzene) and are insoluble in water. Everyone knows that it is impossible to make grease stains on clothes disappear by washing them with water. Instead, they need dry cleaning, using petrol or other grease solvents.

Glycerol (glycerin) is present in abundance in fats. It is a colorless liquid with a syrupy, sweetened taste and is soluble in alcohol.

Lipids constitute the essence of cell membranes. They play a significant role in exchanging molecules from the external world and in their transport within the cell. In the brain, fats constitute the electrical insulation of nerves.

Fats are an essential energy source. All cells can store them, but fat cells store them mainly.

An adult weighing 155 pounds has an energy reserve of 33 pounds of fat, 13 pounds of protein, and 300 grams of carbohydrates (sugars). Seventy-two percent of the remaining weight consists of water. Fatty tissue represents the principal energy reserve of the organism (90 percent).

As noted, food sugar acts immediately. In excess, it can penetrate fat cells, where it can convert sugar into fat. The fat in food is conveyed directly to fatty tissue, contributing to the accumulation of reserves. If the supply of sugary foods is limited, the organism automatically draws on its fat reserves to provide the necessary energy. This mobilization releases glycerol, which is converted to glucose, without which life is impossible. Indeed, whereas other body parts can use various energy sources, the brain permanently consumes *only glucose* (100–150 grams per day). As with a lack of oxygen, a lack of glucose destroys the brain in a few minutes.

The level of sugar in the blood is constant. It results from a balance between the supply of dietary sugar, the synthesis of glycogen by the liver, and its use by the muscles.

This balance is only possible due to hormonal regulation. The traditional conceptualization distinguishes between hormones that raise blood sugar and those that lower it.

Blood sugar levels must imperatively remain constant on an empty stomach. The rise in blood sugar levels caused by food is immediately regulated by insulin, bringing it back to a normal level below 140 milligrams per hundred cubic centimeters of plasma. However, insulin secretion may be insufficient, *leading to* poor glucose metabolism and persistently high blood sugar levels. A simple test can confirm insulin secretion insufficiency. After ingesting seventy-five grams of glucose, the blood sugar must remain lower than or equal to two hundred milligrams per hundred cubic centimeters of plasma (two measurements are necessary). If either measure exceeds 200 milligrams of glucose per hundred cubic centimeters of plasma, the diagnosis of glucose intolerance is possible. This diagnosis can reveal a predisposition to severe disease: diabetes.

When blood sugar exceeds 180 milligrams per hundred cubic centimeters of plasma, glucose molecules are filtered through the renal glomerulus and excreted in the urine.

Ancient writings from Sushruta (six hundred years before Jesus Christ) contain what is probably the first description of diabetes: "When the doctor affirms that the man emits urine comparable with honey, he is declared incurable." In the seventeenth and eighteenth centuries, urine tasters existed; these individuals highlighted the presence of sugar in the urine.

In 1923, Banting and Best discovered insulin, which enabled hormonal control of sugar metabolism, leading to remarkable progress in the treatment of diabetes.

A defect in insulin secretion can occur in young men under 30. Such men suffer from a rare type of abnormal assimilation of sugars, insulin-dependent diabetes, which is determined by hereditary factors

The vast majority of diabetes cases develop after the age of 40 (more than 75 percent), and the frequency of diabetes in the Western population varies between 5 and 25 percent. Many factors contribute to the development of diabetes, but its cause remains poorly defined. Therefore, dietary modification is essential for preventing and treating this severe affliction.

Diabetes causes multiple complications: pruritus (often localized at the genitals), repeated infections, eye troubles (e.g., cataracts), cardiac disorders (e.g., angina pectoris), vascular diseases (e.g., hypertension and gangrene), and nervous disorders (e.g., neuralgias and polyneuritis).

In the United States, diabetes is the third-leading cause of mortality and the number-one cause of blindness. In individuals with diabetes, the coronary risk is multiplied by four. An individual with diabetes older than forty is obese in 80 percent of cases. Premature death from diabetes is directly connected to economic development in various parts of the world. In most countries, diabetes ranks fourth and eighth in causes of mortality.

Classic theories acknowledge a necessary balance between hormones to maintain the constancy of blood sugar levels. Can one ask why the need for *testosterone* is unknown? Testosterone regulates blood sugar levels by allowing glucose to enter the muscles and liver, thereby decreasing blood sugar levels. Conversely, a lack of male hormones raises blood sugar levels.

A permanent lack of testosterone in a man with an androgenic disease of andropause causes a rise in blood sugar. Then there is an immediate consequence: insulin release to bring blood sugar levels back to normal, which provokes a feeling of hunger, commonly called a "need for sugar." The man eats the first food he finds as a preferred source of quick sugars to quickly ease hunger. Again, this provokes an insulin reaction, creating a vicious circle with no end. In men with an androgenic disease of andropause, these phenomena explain the symptoms of excess weight, obesity, and a tendency toward diabetes. It is practically impossible to diet for prolonged periods without an iron will. With the incapacity of doctors to solve the problem, we see the commercial exploitation of weight excess and obesity by charlatans, such as the diffusion of fad diets, which are all claimed to be more effective than others, or by books that are little more than cookbooks.

In 1947, Giuseppe Pellegrini [3] proved that the administration of male hormones decreased the level of blood sugar in individuals with diabetes in an article entitled "The Antidiabetic Action of Male Sex Hormones within the Framework of Diabetes' Physiology" (published in Italian). The clinical study involved 68 patients, including some women. The intramuscular injection of testosterone was found to reduce blood sugar in individuals with diabetes. This reduction occurred gradually, over two or three hours, following the administration of male hormones and lasted until the fourth or fifth hour. The rates of glycosuria decreased simultaneously. The reduction in blood sugar was greater than 1 g/L.

The same phenomenon can be observed in an ordinary man. With him, the blood sugar level does not drop dramatically but remains lower than the average, because his hormonal balance is well-balanced.

In 1984, Ando and colleagues compared the hormonal levels of forty-one diabetics with those of a forty-seven-man reference group with no disease [4]. People with diabetes showed male levels of hormones significantly lower (like older adults' rates) than those of average men.

Insulin acts with remarkable speed. An excess can cause death due to the sharp drop in blood glucose, as the brain has a constant need for glucose. The action of insulin lasts no more than 24 hours, after which blood sugar levels return to their initial values, and new insulin injections are necessary.

Male hormones act more slowly on blood glucose levels. Therefore, when prolonged treatment stops in a person with diabetes, the basal blood sugar (with an empty stomach) returns to the pathological values that preceded the treatment with male hormones.

Male hormones are slow blood sugar regulators, yet their crucial role is ignored. In 1987, Jens Møeller [5], in Copenhagen, confirmed the favorable action of testosterone on diabetic hyperglycemia and glucose intolerance, based on his experience of more than thirty years.

Why Does Man Gain Weight after Forty?

The androgenic disease of andropause (in addition to overeating) is responsible for the vast majority of fatty diabetes and sugar intolerance after age forty. In addition, it causes excess weight and obesity for chemical reasons, worsened by ignorance about good diets.

As noted, the secretion of male hormones decreases after age twenty-five.

Each time sugar enters the blood, it triggers a strong insulin response that stores sugar as fat. The promptness of this reaction goes beyond what is necessary and causes blood sugar levels to fall below average, leading to hunger, discomfort, and a craving for sugar. The vicious cycle is engaged and will develop with time.

No one can break this abnormal cycle without regulating male hormones. Therefore, a man with an androgenic disease of andropause generally cannot control his weight, regardless of his efforts or goodwill. He is always under the influence of discomfort and finally abandons any rational alimentation, which is impossible to sustain over the long term.

As the secretion of male hormones decreases over the years, the abnormal cycle of hyperglycemia, sugar reaction, and insulin release, hunger, and overeating accelerates, leading to excess weight, obesity, and ultimately, death.

In 2001, the National Institute of Health and Medical Research (INSERM) in France demonstrated, in healthy adult men, an improvement in insulin sensitivity with androgen administration [6]. This fascinating study demonstrated the efficacy of androgens in men to correct blood sugar in people with diabetes, emphasizing the importance of dihydrotestosterone.

In 2012, a study published in the *Korean Journal of Family Medicine* examined a population of 388 men aged 40 or older. It showed the correlation between high blood sugar (with an empty stomach) and low testosterone levels in the blood of nondiabetics and prediabetics [7].

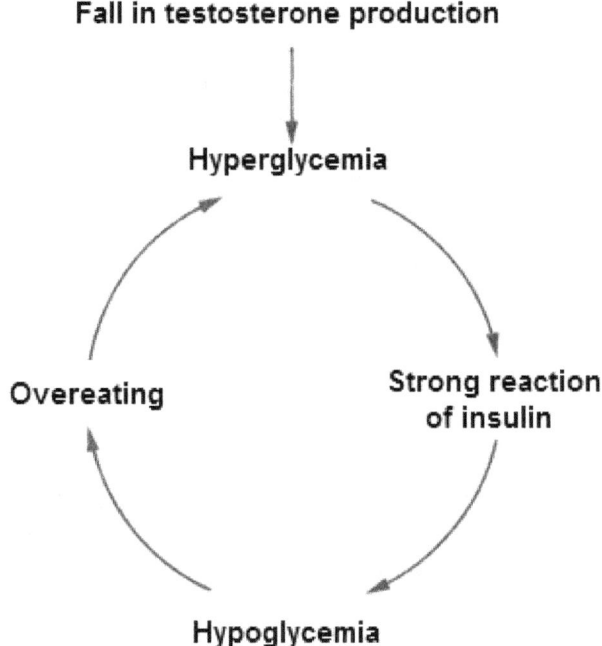

Fig. 11

The abnormal glucose cycle occurs when insulin secretion is sufficient (simplified diagram).

Male Hormones against Cholesterol

> Scientific studies on cholesterol are numerous and continuously evolving. This chapter simply draws attention to *one mechanism* of increased cholesterol in the blood with age: the lack of male hormones, which induce glucose elevation and, consequently, a rise in blood cholesterol.

Poor combustion of sugar and unbalanced food intake produce two well-known phenomena of age: accumulation of cholesterol and fats (triglycerides) in the blood. Measuring cholesterol and blood triglycerides is part of the classic medical checkup. Everyone has heard about the cholesterol of one's grandfather or the triglycerides of one's grandmother. There is no day when the medical press does not call for controlling the rise in blood fats, which increases cardiovascular risk.

It is probably Poulletier de la Salle who isolated, in 1769, the first well-defined lipid, cholesterol, present in gallstones.

In the United States, sixteen to twenty million individuals have gallstones, made up of 80 percent cholesterol. Autopsies showed that at least 8 percent of men had gallstones, and at least 20 percent of women. Each year, one million new cases appear.

Cholesterol comes partly from food, but the liver produces the majority. Its excess in the blood expresses a self-destruction mechanism inherent to the organism.

Fat is a source of energy. Cholesterol in excess is accumulated and stored by the body; its elimination is done almost exclusively by the liver, which excretes it in the bile, where it can crystallize in the form of gallstones.

The balance between cholesterol entry and exit is essential to maintaining the constancy of the interior medium. If there are more entries than needed, cholesterol accumulates in the arteries, and fat deposits under the skin (xanthomas) form.

Cholesterol is primarily produced by the liver. However, food is a secondary source of cholesterol; the intestines absorb only 40 percent of it. These characteristics explain why a diet, regardless of its type, cannot cause a significant drop in blood cholesterol, as the intestines absorb relatively little.

Cholesterol plays a central role in the human body. It participates in the formation of cellular membranes, for example.

It starts with the cholesterol molecule, which the suprarenal glands and testicles use to manufacture hormones (steroids). The action of testosterone, the hormone of construction, is permanently opposed by cortisol. Testosterone increases the synthesis of proteins from the Greek *protos*, which means "first." Proteins are essential substances for the organism. They have exceptional biological properties.

Cortisol, secreted by the adrenal glands, decreases protein synthesis. Testosterone lowers blood sugar levels; cortisol raises them. It is enough to understand that these two hormones act in opposite directions.

Cholesterol is an alcohol in its free state in the organism's cells, where it serves as a precursor for hormones and components of cellular membranes. It also has the property of retaining water within the cells and preventing desiccation. Manufactured by the liver, it is moved toward the organism's cells.

In the plasma, 80% of cholesterol is associated with fatty acids. The "bad" cholesterol is deposited in the form of fats in the arterial walls when it is in excess in the blood.

Fats are insoluble in water. To be transported in the blood, which is aqueous, they bind to proteins (lipoproteins), whose properties enable them to circulate.

Low-density lipoprotein (LDL), a specific lipoprotein, transports the *bad cholesterol*.

"Good" cholesterol is not bound to fatty acids; it is not fat. Instead, it comes from the combustion of unhealthy cholesterol, released of its fatty acids, and represents 27 percent of the total cholesterol in a man aged twenty to twenty-four. A specific lipoprotein, high-density lipoprotein (HDL), transports cholesterol from sites where it is in excess to the liver, where it is degraded and excreted as bile acids.

The rise in blood cholesterol levels also depends on a range of factors beyond the scope of this book.

An increase in blood cholesterol with age in the same population, with the same dietary habits, poses the problem of a fundamental cause that becomes more pronounced over time.

The lipid research program of the National Institutes of Health in the United States defines the average cholesterol level in the population. These results were derived from values determined in eleven communities [1].

Table 4 shows that the rise in blood cholesterol primarily starts with bad cholesterol (LDL cholesterol). It is the bad cholesterol that increases with age. There is a storage of toxic fats. The cause of this accumulation of bad cholesterol is the abnormal cycle of sugar combustion, started by the insufficiency of male hormone secretion in men after age twenty-five.

A lack of male hormones leads to excess sugar, which in turn promotes the synthesis of bad cholesterol because the organism's capacity to eliminate cholesterol is limited.

The accumulation of bad cholesterol results from two different but complementary phenomena. The first is overeating, which increases the glucose contribution. The second is the continued production of cholesterol from excess glucose. Bad cholesterol that is not sufficiently eliminated deposits in the arterial walls.

Average Values of Blood Cholesterol According to Age in the United States			
Age	Total Plasma Cholesterol in mg/100 mL	Plasma LDL Cholesterol in mg/100 mL	Plasma HDL Cholesterol in mg/100 mL
20–24	162	103	45
25–29	179	117	45
30–34	193	126	46
35–39	201	133	43
40–44	205	136	44
45–49	213	144	45
50–54	213	142	44

Table 4

From the US National Institutes of Health [1].

Triglycerides (Fats)

Triglycerides are stored as a reserve substance by specialized cells, adipocytes. They are found under the skin, around abdominal organs in a kind of fatty apron (epiploon) covering the intestines, and in many areas of (obese individuals suffer less from cold than thin people) and protect the organism.

These fats act as heat insulators, protecting the body against shocks. Triglycerides are a reserve of energy.

These reserves are fuel for the organism. They are transported remotely to be "burned" where they are necessary (thanks to very-low-density lipoprotein [VLDL], which also conveys a small portion of bad cholesterol).

Triglyceride levels practically double between twenty and fifty years of age in the fat mass of humans. Therefore, in a study of a population with a similar dietary lifestyle, one can suspect the presence of a fundamental cause that accentuates its harmful effects with age.

The accumulation of triglycerides (fats) is similar to that which determines cholesterol accumulation. However, it acts twice: initially, it collects glucose via an abnormal cycle, and then converts it into triglycerides via acetyl-CoA. Triglycerides accumulate in fat tissue for a long time as food supplies remain excessive.

Many scientific studies have shown the favorable effects of male hormones on cholesterol and triglyceride levels. Good cholesterol (HDL) is higher in men's blood with raised levels of male hormones [2,3].

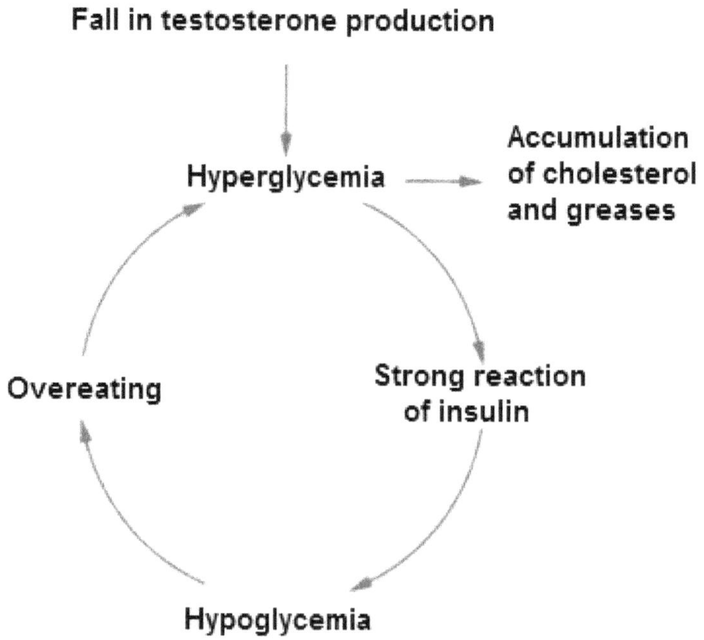

```
         Fall in testosterone production
                        |
                        ↓
                                           Accumulation
              Hyperglycemia  ────────▶     of cholesterol
                                           and greases
                                      
                                      ↓
                              Strong reaction
         Overeating             of insulin
              ↑
               \
                 
              Hypoglycemia
```

Fig. 12

Accumulation of cholesterol and fats in a man with an androgenic disease of andropause (simplified diagram).

Blood triglyceride levels depend on fat reserves and the mobilization of dietary fat. The National Institutes of Health in the United States determined average triglyceride levels by age [1], as shown in Table 5.

A lack of male hormones causes sugar intolerance and diabetes, and dangerously raised levels of cholesterol and fats, thus creating an increase in fat mass and obesity, all of which support the appearance of cardiovascular disease, the leading cause of mortality globally.

Average Triglyceride Levels in Plasma According to Age	
Age	Triglycerides in mg/100 mL
20–24	89
25–29	104
30–34	122
35–39	141
40–44	152
45–49	143
50–54	154

Table 5

Blood triglyceride levels rise with age [1].

Bad cholesterol (LDL-C) is higher in men with low levels of male hormones [5]. Conversely, triglycerides (fat greases) are lower when male hormone levels are high [4,5]. Therefore, low levels of male hormones are directly associated with the rise in blood triglycerides.

Atheroma

Atheroma is sometimes also called *atherosclerosis*. However, the latter term can cause confusion with *arteriosclerosis*, a distinct pathology (see chapter 14). One should not confuse atherosclerosis (atheroma) and arteriosclerosis. *Atheroma* is an entirely relevant term.

In 1904, Marchand coined the term *atherosclerosis—"atheroma"* means "mash" in Greek—to describe the fatty and fibrous degeneration. However, eminent authorities contested this term.

Today, doctors regard atherosclerosis as an entity. Atheroma is the "atheromatous" form of arteriosclerosis—a pathology in which the mechanism is different from *arteriosclerosis* (chapter 14).

Localizations of Atheroma

Atheroma develops in specific locations, depending on the localization of fat deposits, which appear as fatty streaks, fibrous plates, or complex lesions.

Fatty scratches appear, initially characterized by the accumulation of fats, mainly the cholesterol oleate, in the smooth muscle cells and by the development of fibrous tissue under the internal tunic of the artery. These deposits are visible to the naked eye and can appear in any arterial network. Fatty traces are present in the aorta from an early age. At twenty-five years of age, they sometimes occupy 30 to 50 percent of the surface of the aorta. The greasy deposits could reabsorb at this stage, but nothing makes it possible to affirm this.

The fibrous plates appear between the ages of 30 and 40, and their number increases gradually. They develop primarily in the aorta, the heart, the carotid arteries, and the arteries that feed the brain. They consist of a core of fats, principally linoleic acid, and the waste of dead cells, surrounded by many smooth muscle cells and collagen. The whole protrudes into the artery, creating turbulent zones in the bloodstream.

The complicated lesion is a plate encrusted with calcium, containing waste tissue and forming ulcers. While developing, it can completely obliterate the artery (stricture) and serve as the source of an embolism, starting with fragments detached and carried by the bloodstream. In addition, a weakened, thin arterial wall can rupture, leading to internal bleeding.

The increase in fibrous plates and their complications with age pose the problem of a cause that worsens over time.

The Mechanism of Atheroma

The abnormal cycle of glucose excess causes the overproduction of triglycerides and cholesterol in the blood (chapters 10 and 11). Cholesterol in excess cannot be excreted from the body. Instead, when accompanied by fats, it diffuses along the internal walls of the arteries, preferring zones of blood turbulence, such as the aortic crossroads. Consequently, it contacts the elastin fibers. This protein, by its structure, has a strong affinity for fats and calcium. As a result, the elastic structures load cholesterol, fats, and calcium, losing elasticity. The evolution of this process leads to the formation of atheroma.

It is already too late once an atheroma forms, but one can still improve what remains healthy in the arteries. It is necessary to prevent atheroma formation at the early stages of the disease by avoiding the accumulation of harmful cholesterol and fats. We saw the crucial role of male hormones and the need for rigorous food control in this regulation. One does not go without the other.

Control of one's nutrition is fundamental. For example, eating too many sugary and fatty foods and a lack of exercise can cause the formation of atheromas. Individual variations in the production of male hormones clarify sexual differences between individuals. They also explain why some individuals develop atheroma earlier than others.

In 1997, Hoffman and his collaborators showed that atherosclerosis is significantly associated with vascular dementia and Alzheimer's disease (chapter 29) by measuring the relationship between the blood pressures in the arms and the ankles in a group of 284 people with dementia; the thickness of the carotid artery walls was determined by ultrasound [6].

12

Excess Weight and Obesity:

The Ideal Weight

Impaired sugar and cholesterol mechanisms and overeating lead to overweight and obesity. Being overweight, caused by the accumulation of fats, starts with the first extra kilo. At first, this phenomenon is hardly perceptible. But over time, the silhouette changes, kilo by kilo.

Excess weight gradually leads to obesity when the overload reaches 20% of body mass. The obesity of men is characteristic. Fat settles initially in the buttocks, then in the belly, and then gradually invades the top of the body.

The trunk and the shoulders thicken, and then the neck, the nape, and the face. The round, fatty face loses its expressivity because the fat-covered mimetic muscles are unable to move. In addition, fat deposits in the lateral eyelids are characteristic, giving a false impression of sleepiness.

Obesity is a symptom, like a fever. Major metabolic disorders explain certain rare cases of obesity (the huge ones). In most cases, however, the cause of being overweight is unknown, demonstrating the multiple therapeutic attempts, sometimes discouraging, that opened the field to charlatans. The phenomenon reaches worrying proportions in the United States and constitutes a real public health problem worldwide. In terms of obesity frequency, the numbers speak for themselves. According to the World Health Organization (WHO), worldwide, the number of obesity cases has doubled since 1980.

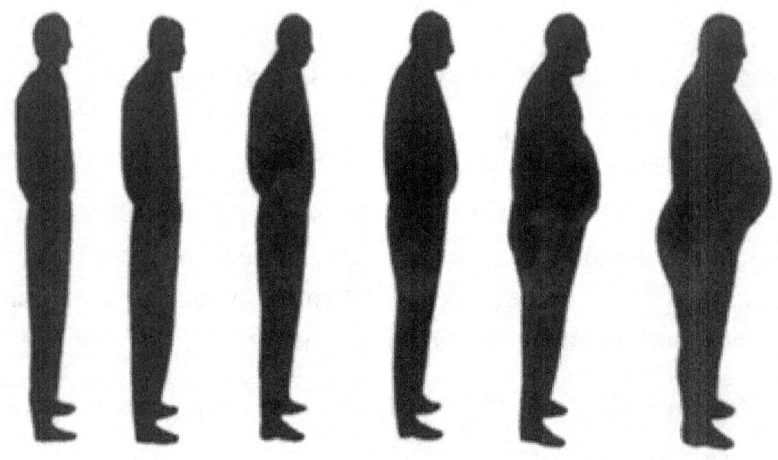

Fig. 13

Outline of a regressive man: age twenty, twenty-five, thirty, forty, forty-five, and fifty-five.

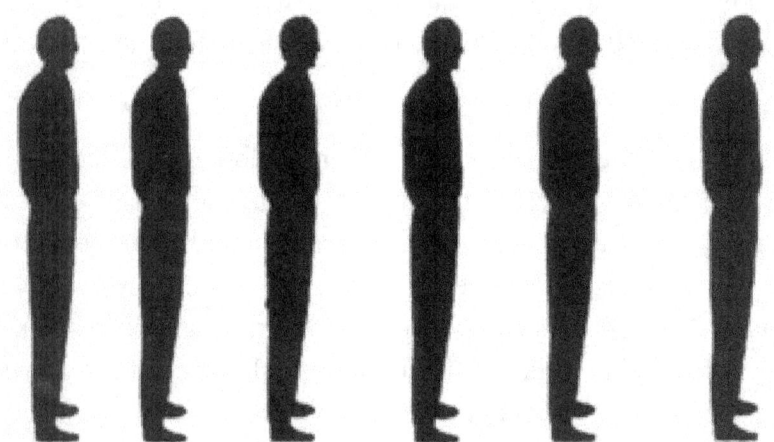

Fig. 14

Outline of an ageless man: twenty to hundred-twenty years.

In 2014, 1.9 billion overweight individuals were eighteen years old or older. Of this total, six hundred million were obese (11 per cent of men and 15 per cent of women). Obesity affects nearly 41 million children under five years of age. According to the WHO, obesity is avoidable.

In the United States, 30 to 40 per cent of the population is overweight by more than 10 per cent. This percentage increases year by year, posing a challenge for the US government, which has invested in extensive research programs to prevent the catastrophe. Obesity accounts for 1 to 3 per cent of total health care costs in most countries (5 to 10 per cent in the United States). The costs will quickly increase in the years to come because obesity increases with diseases of ageing.

Life insurance companies outline clear guidelines on obesity. The Metropolitan Life Insurance Company, for example, published weight tables fixing obesity at an increased body mass of 20 per cent compared to an average person of the same sex and size.

Because the mortality of an obese man is more likely than that of a man having an ideal weight, he pays increased premiums on life insurance. The comparatively high death rate of those who are obese is worrying. Severely obese men die eight to ten years earlier than those with a standard weight, just like smokers. Thirty-three pounds of additional weight increases the risk of premature death by approximately 30 per cent.

What Are the Classifications of Overweight and Obese?

Being overweight or obese is an abnormal or excessive accumulation of body fat, which can harm health.

How does one determine an excess of weight? There are several formulas for determining whether someone is overweight based on body size. None is perfect because individuals differ constitutionally (e.g., a man with solid bones and musculature is more massive). One of the most recent is the body mass index (BMI). This index divides the weight in kilograms by the height squared, expressed in meters.

$$BMI = \frac{Weight\ (kilos)}{H^2\ (meters)}$$

The WHO defines overweight and obesity as follows:

- Overweight is a BMI equal to or higher than twenty-five.
- Obese is a BMI equal to or higher than thirty.

In 1959, the ideal weight tables of the Metropolitan Life Insurance Company corresponded to a BMI of 22; above 22 was considered overweight.

It is necessary to receive appropriate treatment to avoid exceeding this index level. Correction of weight is more feasible at the early stage of fat accumulation. It has even been said that an average excess of two pounds shortens one's life by two months.

What Is Your Ideal Weight?

One should consider the BMI formula to answer this question. The formula is as follows:

22 ′ height (in meters)2 = ideal weight

For example, for a height of 1.80 meters: 22 ′ 1.822 = 22 ′ 3.24 = 71.28 kilos (157.14 pounds) = ideal weight.

Thinness is also not a good sign. Lew and Garfinkel [1] showed, in a study relating to a population of 750,000 men and women, a higher death rate of individuals whose weight was lower than 10 percent of the standard weight.

However, remaining thin due to a suitable diet does not mean the same. Some even recommend systematic malnutrition to increase longevity. This approach could be considered, provided it is not misused to lead to thinness*

Energy reserves are necessary to fight disease and support a fasting period. Whatever the diet, it must be balanced to maintain the proper weight because obesity causes devastation.

Complications, whose frequency is well known, reduce the longevity of the obese.

What Are the Most Frequent Consequences of Being Overweight or Obese?

A high BMI is a significant risk factor for chronic diseases, such as the following:

• Cardiovascular disease (mainly heart disease and stroke), which is the leading cause of death worldwide

• Diabetes

• Muscular and skeletal disorders (e.g., osteoarthritis, a degenerative disease of the joint articulations)

• Certain cancers (e.g., of the endometrium, breast, and colon)

Fat mass doubles between the ages of 18 and 50, and continues to increase thereafter. At the same time, muscular mass decreases.

---

* Thinness is the result of the disappearance, reduction, or insufficiency of the fat reserves of the organism, sometimes accompanied by atrophy of the muscular masses.

Simple observation makes this possible. We know that testosterone secretion decreases after age twenty-five. This hormone is necessary for maintaining muscularity and fat mass. Bringing these phenomena together clarifies the cause and consequences (other factors worsen the situation).

A progressive lack of male hormones can cause one to become overweight, which increases with age. All therapeutic efforts generally relate to the diet, particular foods, and general measures. Nevertheless, the prevalence of obesity continues to increase worldwide. In individuals, it develops with time (figure 13, page 116).

Admittedly, some men maintain their weight within reasonable limits through a balanced diet and exercise, driven by willpower. But not all men have an iron will. Discouragement and relapses are the rules despite the desire to lose weight.

Old, frustrated, obese men often deploy ingenuity and diet-program calculations, generally without result. Why this frustration? Men under twenty usually eat anything and do not gain weight because they have a maximum secretion of male hormones (figure 14, page 116).

Male hormones cause the mobilization of reserve fats (lipolysis). The mechanism is complex and is beyond the scope of this text.

Clinical studies showed a decrease in male hormones in the obese. In 1990, Zumoff and his collaborators confirmed a reduction in the plasma-free testosterone and total testosterone levels in the obese. The drop in the plasma level was proportional to obesity [2].

The human organism is perpetually in a balance between construction and destruction. The treatment of obesity is, overall, a failure. The regulation of hormones is vital to maintaining the body's stability. However, chemistry cannot do everything. The following is important: we are not obligated to eat four times a day (or more!). In managing weight, it is necessary to ensure calm for the brain.

It is illogical to think that food restrictions alone can suffice to ensure longevity. It is essential to reinforce the construction of the out-of-date fatty organism, which breaks down thanks to testosterone, the structure hormone.

In 2009, a scientific study showed a significant reduction in waist measurement in men presenting hypogonadism after fifty-two weeks of treatment with diet, exercise, and a gel of testosterone on the skin [3].

Many doctors associate testosterone treatment with prostate cancer or cardiovascular disease risk. These "beliefs" have no foundation (see chapter 9). Worse, they are the opposite of reality and condemn millions of human beings to develop ageing diseases.

According to a study by Farid Saad and his collaborators, obesity treatment is, overall, a failure. This study showed in 2012 that testosterone's favorable action in treating obesity [4]. In cases of androgenic disease of andropause (see Chapter 1), initial therapy with mesterolone should be considered based on biological data and before starting testosterone therapy (see Chapter 33).

13

Muscular Weakness

Muscle contracts due to the energy provided by sugar and glycogen, which are muscle fuels. It is a complex molecule used as an energy reserve. Subunits of glucose make glycogen an essential source of energy for the body. One finds it in honey, grapes, and fruits.

Blood sugar levels depend on the quantity of ingested sugar and its release from muscle and liver reserves—even fat tissue stores glucose in the form of fatty acids and triglycerides.

In a healthy state, there is a balance between blood glucose levels and the reserves stored in muscles and fat.

With an empty stomach, the average blood sugar level is lower than 140 milligrams per hundred cubic centimeters of venous blood (two measurements are necessary to confirm constancy of the disordered state beyond 140) [1], with the ideal being around one hundred.

If one translates these milligrams into molecules[*] that represents a billion molecules in circulation. Blood makes a complete turn through the organism in one minute; blood flow in organs is thus extremely high. For example, a healthy kidney contains 100 billion cells. One liter, or 200 cubic centimeters, of blood irrigates this organ in one minute. So, in each minute, several billion glucose molecules penetrate each cell [2].

This phenomenon is similar in the muscles, which permanently receive considerable amounts of glucose, which is then transformed and stored as glycogen. Without it, muscles do not function, just as a car cannot

---

[*] The molecule is the smallest particle of matter that preserves its characteristics.

run without gasoline. Glycogen is a muscle's fuel. It is permanently "burned" at the time of the muscular contraction.

The effects of male hormones on muscle tissue have been known for many years. First, male hormones enter the muscle cell, where they bind to a specific receptor, as shown by Jung and Beaulieu [3] and other authors. Next, the hormone moves toward the cell nucleus, starting its hormonal effect. The essential reactions are of two types. Initially, protein synthesis increases by incorporating new amino acids (the subunits of proteins). Then, glycogen contents also increase significantly [4]. Hypertrophy of the muscle follows, as is well known by athletes who wish to improve their performance. The consumption of male hormones increases during physical exercise. Blood testosterone drops during prolonged efforts.

Plas [5] studied the evolution of testosterone and dihydrotestosterone levels before and after an effort in eleven voluntary athletes. Three days without interruption, they were subjected to two daily cyclists' tests of two and a half hours each, conducted at a mean velocity of forty kilometers per hour, interspersed with rest. This study showed a reduction in the male hormone rate that persisted for 4 days after the effort ended. It is necessary to wait 10 days to restore hormonal secretion before the action.

Blood testosterone drops in athletes after a race of one hundred kilometers [6]. This test consists of covering 100 kilometers in a 24-hour period. It takes place day and night, alone or in a group, in the sun or rain, at any temperature, in conditions that demand physical effort. The study team consists of fourteen runners aged twenty-eight to forty-five. All present on arrival with a significant reduction in blood testosterone. The testosterone level in blood increases five days after the start of the race and peaks around the ninth day.

In an athlete, prolonged effort increases the consumption of male hormones. Excessive use of male hormones during protracted physical efforts causes a lowering of the blood levels of male hormones, resulting in two principal consequences. The first is psychological. The drop in the testosterone level in the blood causes a feeling of tiredness and depression, increasing with effort, leading finally to abandonment. The second is metabolic. The drop in blood testosterone prevents the muscle's energy stores from recovering. The fuel (glycogen) is missing—avoiding any extra effort, the athlete crumbles, unable to move.

The lack of male hormones also causes serious heart diseases. Many young men die from sudden deaths during sports. From 1974 to 1977, seventeen cases of sudden deaths during cyclists' competitions were reported in professional athletes in excellent health who were chosen for the race through strict selection [7].

In 2013, researchers in the Department of Endocrinology, Diabetes, and Nutrition at Boston Medical Center demonstrated that testosterone promotes skeletal muscle regeneration in castrated mice [8]. Cellular regeneration and cell proliferation were evident four days after castration in young, two-month-old mice, as in old, twenty-four-month-old mice.

An excess of male hormones increases the muscular mass beyond what is reasonable. The opposite is also exact: a lack of male hormones causes a reduction in the muscular mass and its atrophy*. Muscles, motility agents, are atrophied in men with an androgenic disease of andropause. An increase in fat and a decrease in muscular mass transform the body, making it soft rather than firm. This fact leads to a reduction in the density of older adults. Body density varies from 1,040

---

* Atrophy is characterized by a reduction in the volume of a living structure caused by inadequate nutrition, disuse, a physiological process of regression, or disease.

at around twenty to 1,016 at approximately fifty years. The weakened musculature of older adults is an indication of androgen therapy.

The physical effort of the man with the androgenic disease of andropause has increasingly large limits over time. Deprived of male hormones, he is less and less competitive. In tennis, young people defeat him. Elsewhere, he still lags. High-level sporting events are unfair to men over 25. Deprived of male hormones, they cannot win against young people, who naturally produce high quantities of male hormones. It explains why it is practically impossible for a forty-year-old to win the Olympic Games. One cannot prevent oneself from quivering while thinking of the older adults who launch excessive efforts to prove they still exist. It can be observed that in gyms, after exercise, men with androgenic andropause present greyish, fatigued faces. They should support their physical effort by taking male hormones. During a famous marathon, it frequently happens that an older man crumbles and dies who, in any event, had an androgenic disease of andropause. All in all, it was a race with a lost body.

14

Arteriosclerosis or Arterial Rigidity

You are as old as your arteries

Arteriosclerosis, also known as *arterial rigidity, is a common condition.* Webster's New World College Dictionary defines it as "arteriosclerosis, an abnormal thickening and loss of elasticity of arterial walls. *Origin of arteriosclerosis* (arterio- + sclerosis)." But dictionaries sometimes give another definition that confuses *arteriosclerosis* with *atherosclerosis*. Healthy arteries are flexible and elastic, but the walls of arteries can harden over time, a condition commonly called *hardening of the arteries*, which sometimes restricts blood flow to organs and tissues.

Warning

Arteriosclerosis is a specific pathology, whereas *atherosclerosis* is a different concept.

The definition of the 2016 edition of the *American Heritage Dictionary of the English Language* is as follows:

Atherosclerosis is a form of arteriosclerosis characterized by lesions (called plaques) in the innermost layer of the walls of large and medium-sized arteries. The plates contain lipids, collagen, inflammatory cells, and other substances and can impede blood flow or rupture, leading to severe problems such as a heart attack or stroke.

The term *atherosclerosis* was invented one day by an enlightened mind that confounded two arterial pathologies: the first caused by sclerosis of arterial walls, and the second by deposits of greasy plates. In the first case, it is a disease. In the latter case, it is a syndrome (chapter 11).

Arteriosclerosis is a disease of ageing with a specific cause, consequences, and a particular treatment. In the medical literature, the causes of arteriosclerosis remain unknown. However, the cause is as follows.

Pathological cuts of a sclerosed artery show disorganization of muscle fibers and their replacement by rigid fibrous tissue (the tissue of scars). Arterial resistance to blood-wave propagation increases, leading to hypertension upstream of the functional obstacle. The internal wall of the artery, subjected to a permanent excess of pressure, thickens, reducing the arterial diameter.

Arteriosclerosis is the keystone of cardiovascular disease. It constitutes the first cause of mortality in Western countries and the US [1].

Before age sixty-five, men die more frequently from the complications of arteriosclerosis than women; after this age, degeneration strikes women as much as men.

Arteriosclerosis is a common phenomenon after age forty. It is the leading cause of mortality after age sixty-five. The eighty-year-old man generally presents with signs of arteriosclerosis. The expression "you are as old as your arteries" is significant here.

Mechanism of Arteriosclerosis

The mechanism of arteriosclerosis differs from that of atheroma (chapter 11). Why do arteries harden with age?

For some authors, arteriosclerosis is a typical degenerative process that accompanies ageing; it is not a disease. This degeneration is not influenced by risk factors. Others call upon the importance of diet, fats in blood, and the role of cigarette smoking, psychic stress, and other factors that can interact with the pathogenesis of arteriosclerosis. These elements, however, do not seem to explain the origin of arterial hardening. Hypertension, age-related factors, and constitutional factors have also been cited to explain arteriosclerosis. For many people, the cause of arteriosclerosis remains a mystery.

One element must draw our attention. Histological sections of sclerosed arteries can reveal certain features. The pathologist will observe, without difficulty, that the lesions of arterial walls show characteristics of scar tissue. In arteriosclerosis, the connective tissue replaces the muscle fibers. But what is the cause?

Muscular arteries regulate arterial flow [2]. Therefore, they constitute a real engine necessary for the propulsion of blood waves.

Proteins and glycogen are energetic factors required to run this engine. However, muscle fibers are less contractile when dynamic contributions decrease, becoming progressively weaker over time. As a result, they die, replaced by fibrous tissue containing rigid collagen, unable to propagate the blood wave.

The comparison with the ureter, a conduit whose motility depends on its musculature, seems evident to me. The ureter, whose muscle fibers have been replaced by sclerosed tissue, cannot propel urine. In the same circumstances, the artery will not be able to move the blood.

After nine years of study in a university pathology laboratory, I observed, in 1971, a comparable phenomenon in the ureteral wall at the point where it enters the bladder (the terminal ureter) [3, 4]. At that time, I wondered why some children presented with ureters that were very dilated (megaureter) without an apparent cause. Urine accumulated in the dilated ureter and crossed with difficulty in its final segment, not seemingly narrowed. The phenomenon was often attributed to hypothetical nervous disorders. This anomaly involved the destruction of the kidneys, invariably caused by hypertension in the ureter. I compared the healthy structure of the normal terminal ureter with that of segments unable to propagate the wave of urine in a pathological study involving more than 50,000 histological sections. In all cases, the musculature of the final ureter was defective, or the seat of malformations, and was replaced, generally by rigid fibrous tissue unable to propagate the urinary wave [3, 4].

When a segment of the ureter is sclerosed, it results in an upstream overload. As a result, the ureter dilates above the obstacle. Its muscle fibers, subjected to excessive work, hypertrophy initially. Over time, these fibers become atrophied and are replaced by fibrous tissue within the dilated ureter [5].

The phenomenon is similar in arteries, where smooth muscle fibers act as an engine that propels the blood wave.

Extra work is required in the upstream arterial musculature when an arterial segment becomes fibrous anywhere in the arterial network. As a result, it hypertrophies initially and then atrophies mechanically. Additionally, the muscle fibers of the entire arterial musculature degenerate due to a lack of energy factors.

The arterial muscular engine, like any engine, cannot function without the contribution of energy in the form of proteins and glycogen.

The conjunctive tissue between the arterial muscle fibers also becomes rigid due to the lack of male hormones (chapter 19).

Mesterolone normalizes the structure of muscle fibers. Under these conditions, arterial stiffness will not occur with ageing. Therefore, there will be no hypertension. And if there is no hypertension, no antihypertensive treatment will be necessary [6].

Arteriosclerosis is consequently the result of the following:

1. Degeneration of the muscle fibers of the artery from a lack of male hormones, thus preventing the incorporation of energy factors like proteins and glycogen in the arterial musculature

2. A rigidity of conjunctive arterial tissue from a lack of male hormones

3. An excess of pressure on the walls of the artery upstream from a rigid fibrous segment anywhere in the arterial network, causing the mechanical hypertrophy of the arterial musculature and then its atrophy

and its replacement by fibrous tissue, in addition to its biological degeneration (see points 1 and 2).

Those consequences are a perfect example of the vicious pathological cycles that imply several pathogeneses.

All women and men are eventually affected by arteriosclerosis, as hormonal production gradually decreases with age.

The energy substrates (proteins and glycogen) suddenly disappear from the arterial muscular structures. They degenerate quickly, replaced by rigid fibrous tissue. Consequently, the tiny arteries at the end of the arterial network do not regularly supply blood to organs, including the eyes, ears, and hippocampus, in Alzheimer's disease (chapter 29).

Doctors are confronted daily with the devastations of cardiovascular disease. An aspect of prevention involves supervising patients' cholesterol levels and prescribing cholesterol-lowering drugs. They could improve their patients' health by also managing male hormones when necessary. A man with "good" biological results with his cholesterol under cholesterol-lowering drugs will inevitably develop arteriosclerosis due to a lack of male hormones.

The male hormone is a general concept that does not explain "what to do" and "how to do it." For example, testosterone is an androgen, but it is an anabolic hormone that needs to be converted into another one to be androgenic.

In *Merriam-Webster's* definition, an androgenic hormone is a steroid hormone, such as testosterone, that controls the development and maintenance of masculine characteristics. In this definition, the term *control* has a general meaning. Therefore, a better description would be: "an androgenic hormone is a steroid hormone, such as testosterone, that could influence the development and maintenance of masculine characteristics." However, this definition is also too general.

In a man of age twenty, testosterone and dihydrotestosterone are well balanced. However, when production declines with ageing, for technical reasons, testosterone and dihydrotestosterone, which are then artificial hormones, may not be introduced into the body without provoking a biological disturbance [6]. Therefore, they are not approved for use in women by the US Food and Drug Administration (FDA) for good reason.

The FDA is still extremely cautious about the use of testosterone in men. The current content of the FDA as of 02/26/2018 is—FDA Drug Safety Communication: FDA cautions about using testosterone products for low testosterone due to ageing; it requires labeling change to inform of possible increased risk of heart attack and stroke with use.

> The FDA could be even more cautious. Testosterone is not the treatment for the androgenic disease of andropause (chapter1). Likely, many cases of Low Testosterone do not require testosterone treatment but rather a cautious and safe supplementation with mesterolone (chapter1).

An eighty-year-old man treated with mesterolone for forty years has no arteriosclerosis nor hypertension [6]. Therefore, he can continue his treatment indefinitely without any danger of being treated with mesterolone, thus preventing many diseases of ageing (see part II).

The body of a man not treated since the age of forty is almost destroyed at the age of eighty. In some cases, treatment with androgens is formally contraindicated.

Thus, artificial testosterone and dihydrotestosterone are inappropriate and not valid for preventing arteriosclerosis.

Diseases of ageing progress to permanent vascular disorders due to arteriosclerosis. The tiny arteries that constitute the end of the arterial network are particularly vulnerable. They are the first to have diminished blood flow. Their obstruction deprives the cells of oxygen, causing their destruction. Essential molecules are necessary for the survival of these cells, which are also compromised.

What to Do to Prevent Arteriosclerosis?

The preceding discussion notwithstanding, a solution does exist to prevent arteriosclerosis and its numerous complications, which include the following:

- Arterial hypertension
- Hearing and vision troubles (e.g., cataracts, retinal detachment, age-related macular degeneration)
- Angina pectoris
- Myocardial infarct
- Arterial rupture
- Vascular degeneration of joint articulations
- Renal insufficiency
- Arterial occlusion of the lower extremities
- Parkinson's disease
- Alzheimer's disease
- Stroke

A lack of dihydrotestosterone is the first step in an anabolic hormone deficiency. With mesterolone, a safe molecule, it is possible to substitute the anabolic deficit around age forty or before [6].

Indeed, dihydrotestosterone is the final androgen hormone. Testosterone is a precursor of dihydrotestosterone, just as dehydroepiandrosterone (DHEA) is a precursor of testosterone. Therefore, neither testosterone nor DHEA can replace dihydrotestosterone.

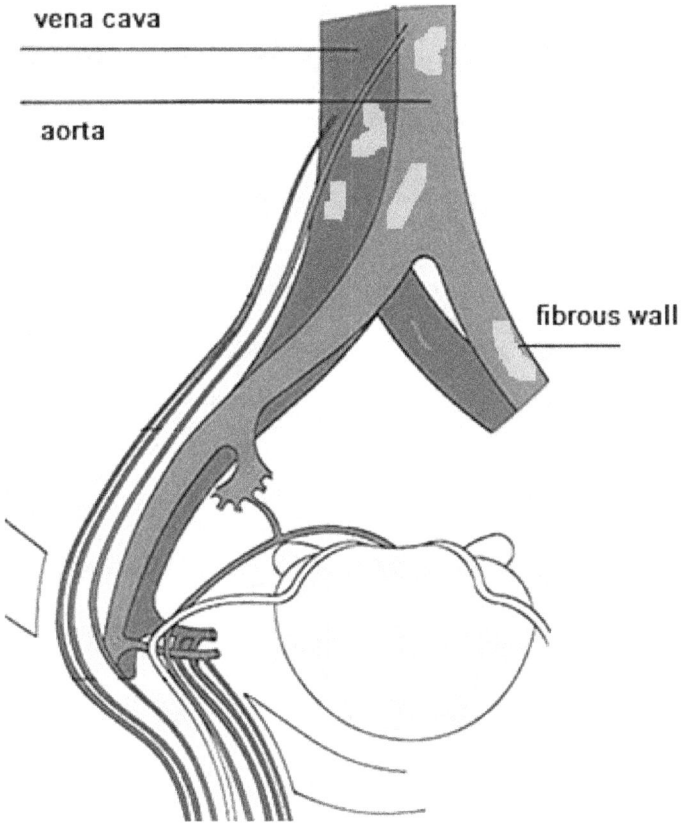

Fig. 15

Figure 15 shows areas at the early stages of degeneration. Degenerating plaques of the aorta and iliac artery are shown in light grey. With age, the number of these fibrous areas will grow, and the fibrous tissue will invade the entire arterial network. The arterial muscle tissue degenerates. A lack of muscle development in men and women leads to muscle degeneration.

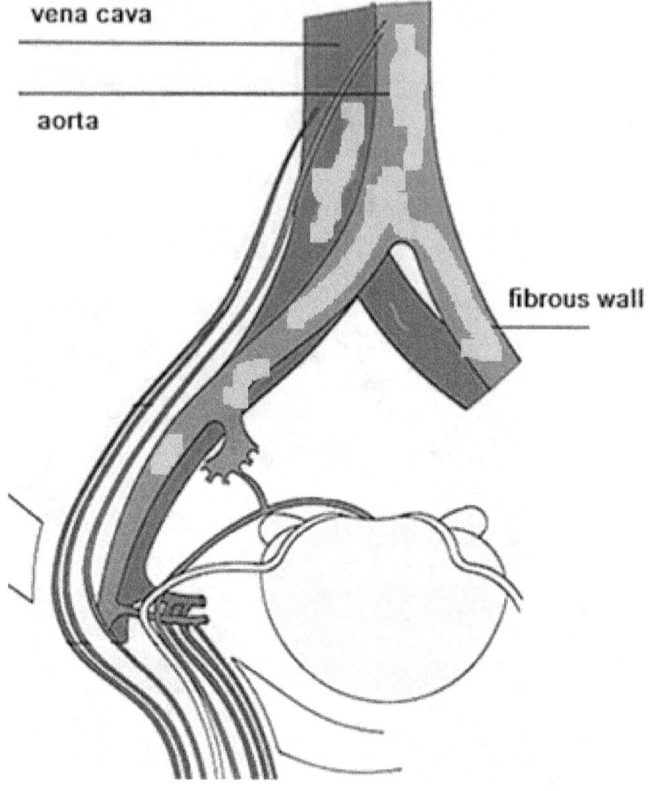

Fig. 16

Arteriosclerosis is a Disease

- It has a cause, a lack of energetic factors for arterial muscle fibers.
- It has a direct consequence: the fibrosis of the arterial muscle. (Figure 16). Fibrous tissue in light grey.
- It has a preventive daily permanent treatment for life with mesterolone from age forty and before [6].

There is an overall lack of androgen production in ageing men and women when dihydrotestosterone is low. Then the global production of anabolic hormones starts to decrease, although the nonsexual functions are, in part, spared.

Heavy testosterone treatments are dangerous for men with low testosterone (i.e., whose *production* of male hormones is almost nonexistent). In this condition, all arterial muscle structures have degenerated for decades, thereby limiting life expectancy to an average of 80 years.

As for women, they do not have an age-dependent treatment for androgens because this need is ignored, *while the healthy woman physiologically produces more testosterone than the female hormone every day.*

However, it is possible to compensate for the lack of anabolism at its inception. It is enough to take mesterolone at the outset of the deficiency, depending on the biochemical dosage characteristics of each individual, who is around forty years of age, and sometimes even before.

Mesterolone is not known as a potent anabolic. Therefore, it is scorned by the medical corps in the treatment of low testosterone syndrome in older men. In contrast, low testosterone medical conditions would not even exist if correct prevention by mesterolone had been done forty years earlier.

Mesterolone is a weak anabolic, which gives it exceptional therapeutic quality. Its anabolic properties are sufficient to maintain the networks of arterial muscle fibers throughout life. It is a hormone for extended, healthy living, a keystone.

In general, mesterolone is prescribed for a few months in men with a deficiency in androgen production. The pharmaceutical industry excluded women from treatment, reasoning that the dosage of tablets sold is suitable for men only. The pharmaceutical industry has not yet realized the potential of mesterolone tablets for women. They would be simple to produce.

However, the prevention of arteriosclerosis must begin around the age of forty years, and sometimes even before, with daily doses taken throughout life. In my experience, three older people over age eighty— a woman and two men—were found to have a blood pressure of 12/8 and even 12/7.5 after several decades of continuous and preventive treatment with mesterolone [6]. After forty, this treatment prevents high blood pressure and all disorders caused or aggravated by arteriosclerosis.

By measuring dihydrotestosterone production, it is possible to compensate for anabolic deficiencies.

Therefore, mesterolone should be the best-selling drug globally because it would benefit everyone [6].

15

Anemia

Red blood cells contain hemoglobin, a protein substance containing iron, and play a crucial role in oxygen transport. Therefore, reducing red blood cell count and hemoglobin content leads to anemia.

The symptoms are paleness, tiredness, breathlessness, pulse acceleration, syncope, giddiness, and digestive disorders. Anemia can result from heavy bleeding (hemorrhage) or a disorder of the red cells caused by infectious or toxic agents. Red blood cells also depend on specific hormones that stimulate their production.

The number of red blood cells in a man varies between 4,500,000 and 5,900,000 per cubic millimeter of blood (the standard can vary by laboratory). Therefore, symptoms of anemia can appear at a red blood cell count below 4,500,000 per cubic millimeter of blood.

The "normal" number of globules is a statistical notion based on the whole adult male population; however, each person is unique. Let us imagine that man's ideal number of red globules is 5,500,000 per cubic millimeter of blood. The doctor will regard a laboratory analysis showing him to have 4,500,000 red globules, within the statistical average, as "normal." However, compared to this same man's ideal number of red globules, he will miss 20 percent of them per cubic millimeter of plasma. It is consequently helpful to know the number of red globules at around twenty years, when the organism is in proper form, and compare it with the blood samples taken during ageing. A fall from 10 to 20 percent of red globules can decrease tissue oxygenation. When the number of red globules approaches 4,500,000, one can wonder whether anemia exists, given that this average seems "normal."

The biological averages, calculated with the whole of an older population, the rates are lower, since the physiological rates of young men become increasingly marginal relative to the "average." At the limit, being a minority, young people would be regarded as "abnormal." It is necessary to pay closer attention to this drift in statistical interpretation.

Medically, imposing this average overall on a population constitutes a severe error, and more, a fault. Each human being is singular and represents a vital force in the whole becoming, worthy of greater respect. Raising a man in this spirit is necessary, not lowering him. Male hormones influence the formation of red globules. Castration in rats produces a fall in male hormones and the appearance of anemia [1]. Kennedy noted, in 1956, that in women presenting advanced breast cancer and suffering from anemia, the number of red globules increased spectacularly, giving them male hormones [2-3].

Many diseases cause anemia. Treatment with male hormones is beneficial in many patients [4]. In 1981, Najean showed that, in a series of 137 patients treated for more than 2 years, anemia worsened with the discontinuation of male hormone therapy and improved when treatment was resumed [5]. Today, one can study the effects of male hormones on cultured bone marrow stem cells. Male hormones activate the stem cells to make red globules [6].

In the castrate, the number of red globules decreases by 10 percent.

The man with an androgenic disease of andropause often presents a reduction of his red blood cells, which increases when taking male hormones.

In 2006, a study published in the *Archives of Internal Medicine* showed a high risk of anemia among men and women presenting low testosterone levels. The Clinical Research Branch, National Institute on Aging of Baltimore, carried out these scientific observations with several scientific centers [7]

16

Viscous Blood, Embolisms, Thromboses, Varicose Veins and Hemorrhoids

Viscous Blood

The formation of a clot is caused by many factors that act successively to initiate a chain reaction, ultimately leading to fibrin, an insoluble fibrillary gel that constitutes the clot. Blood would coagulate in the absence of factors; at the same time, the clot would undergo permanent lysis (fibrinolysis).

Blood contains specific chemical factors that cause coagulation and chemical activators (e.g., antithrombin III) that ensure fluidity. The chemical reactions that start coagulation and those that cause fluidity are complex. The important thing is to know that these forces are in a state of permanent balance.

When coagulation factors are missing, unverifiable hemorrhages sometimes occur. Hemophilia is well known. It is a hereditary disease characterized by a delay of coagulation and disproportionately prolonged hemorrhages that lack the tendency to stop spontaneously. In individuals with hemophilia, even tooth removal constitutes a significant risk. Trauma can cause bleeding in the muscles or the articulations and can be fatal. Fortunately, hemophilia is an uncommon illness.

On the other hand, excessive blood coagulation is widespread after age 60. The factors that determine fluidity cannot ensure normal blood fluidity. Thick blood gives rise to thromboses and embolisms.

Thrombosis

The formation of a clot in a blood vessel can cause occlusion of an artery or a vein.

Arterial thrombosis develops at arterial wall wear points, caused by arteriosclerosis. The arteries of the extremities are most often affected, which can lead to gangrene. Thrombosis of cerebral arteries has severe neurological consequences, such as paralysis.

Venous thrombosis results from slowed blood flow or uncontrolled coagulation. The phenomenon is already worrying when it develops in medium-caliber veins, but it can be fatal in large blood vessels.

Embolisms

The sudden obliteration of a vessel is a serious incident. It results from a clot that detaches from the heart's walls during cardiac failure, or from zones of excessive turbulence at arterial walls, arterial junctions, or atheromas. The abrupt obliteration of a large artery requires urgent surgery under a surgeon specializing in vascular techniques.

Cardiovascular disease is the primary source of thromboses and embolisms. Therefore, many patients permanently take anticoagulant medicines. They must check the fluidity of their blood through repeated blood tests, because these substances must sufficiently lower the coagulation factors to be active. Treatment with anticoagulants is not without risk. Beyond a critical point, a renal, gastric, or cerebral hemorrhage can occur.

The most used anticoagulants are heparin and dicoumarol. Heparin, used in intravenous injections, acts instantaneously. It inhibits the first and second stages of the coagulation cascade.

Dicoumarol, taken orally, works more slowly because it inhibits the vitamin K1 required for the first stage of clotting. Therefore, patients who receive this treatment must permanently monitor their prothrombin times, which should range between 20 and 30 percent. Below that, there is a risk of bleeding.

Dicoumarol prevents blood from coagulating, but does not dissolve the clot, which is done by other molecules. Thick blood results from an incapacity of fluidity factors to create the clot lysis. The patients who have thromboembolic vascular disorders present with a defect of fibrinolysis.

Male Hormones Are Natural Blood Thinners

In 1988, Bonithon-Kopp and colleagues [1] showed that low plasma testosterone levels were associated with hypercoagulability. The same year, Caron and colleagues [2] confirmed that fibrinolysis is an essential system for preventing the development of venous and arterial thromboses and is favorably influenced by male hormones. Other authors prescribed male hormones to thin the blood of patients suffering from vascular disorders [3,4]. By regulating male hormones, the blood becomes thinner due to increased production of antithrombin III (a thinning factor). When treatment is interrupted, the blood becomes thick again due to reduced antithrombin III production. Blood once again becomes fluid with the resumption of androgens.

In conclusion, male hormones are natural factors that enhance blood fluidity by stimulating the production of antithrombin III. Their administration does not pose a bleeding risk, unlike anticoagulants. The World Health Organization recommends treating thromboembolic cardiovascular diseases with testosterone [5].

Antithrombin (also called *antithrombin III* or *AT III*) is a coagulation inhibitor. Therefore, a deficit in antithrombin predisposes to thromboses.

In 2009, a study showed that testosterone administration increased fluidity factors in people with diabetes with foot ulcers [6].

Varicose Veins and Hemorrhoids

Heavy Legs

Varicose veins develop with age, especially in the legs. Superficial veins are dilated, irregular, tortuous, and unsightly in appearance. After a long period in an upright position, they cause a feeling of "heavy legs" that gradually intensifies throughout the day. The feet are swollen due to edema.

Varicose veins can also result from compression of the venous network. This phenomenon is rare in men. In women, who are more predisposed to developing varicose veins, the venous dilations can appear during pregnancy. They become more frequent with obesity and age. Varicose veins can become complicated by varicose phlebitis and ulcers.

Phlebitis is an inflammation of the venous walls. It causes pulmonary embolisms in 5 to 6 percent of cases. Pulmonary embolism represents a significant cause of mortality and results in more than fifty thousand deaths in the United States annually. However, pulmonary embolism is fatal in only 10 percent of cases; thus, one can estimate the annual number of pulmonary embolisms in the US as more than five hundred thousand.

A varicose ulcer is a significant ulceration of the leg, usually caused by chronic venous insufficiency. The loss of skin substance may result from minor trauma, a common cutaneous infection, or the thrombosis of a dilated vein. Varicose ulcers are difficult to cure.

Hemorrhoids

Varicose veins of the anus and rectum create venous tumors called *hemorrhoids*. Like all varicose veins, they can cause inflammation and painful thromboses. External hemorrhoids are located below the anal sphincter and are visible to the naked eye. Internal hemorrhoids located above the anal sphincter are viewable by anoscopy.

In a man with the androgenic disease of andropause, hemorrhoids must bring attention to the existence of prostate hypertrophy that compresses the varicose networks. The large prostate compresses the veins. Removing it before surgery for the hemorrhoid problem can be helpful to get a better result.

Medical books do not explain why venous walls can be weak in humans except for compression phenomena.

Veins, like the arteries, consist of elastic tissues. After irrigating organs, blood returns to the heart via the venous network. Initially, small venules collect blood, then progressively larger veins. The venules continue in the muscular veins of the extremities and internal organs. Some of these veins are strengthened and form a system of pumps that propel blood toward the heart, including the pelvic veins, the large veins of the lower extremities, and the large vena cava.

A lack of male hormones automatically triggers the same regressive transformations observed in arterial wall musculature. As a result, the smooth muscles degenerate, replaced by rigid fibrous tissue. Also, the other elastic components lose their elasticity. These degenerative transformations compromise blood flow. As a result, the return of blood toward the heart is impaired. Excess coagulation is responsible for unexplained phlebitis [7] and certain leg ulcers [8].

Bennet and colleagues [9] showed in 1987 that venous stasis tends to form clots in patients lacking male hormones. This tendency toward thrombosis normalized after three months of treatment with dihydrotestosterone, administered as a cutaneous gel at 125 milligrams per day.

Male hormones are necessary to flex venous walls and ensure blood fluidity.

Hypertension, Disease of the World

According to the World Health Organization (WHO), cardiovascular diseases were responsible for approximately 17 million deaths in the world in 2008—that is to say, nearly a third of the total mortality rate. In addition, 9.4 million deaths yearly are caused by hypertension (high blood pressure) complications. Hypertension is responsible for at least 45 percent of deaths from cardiac diseases and 51 percent of deaths from strokes.

In 2016, hypertension affected nearly one-third of US residents aged 18 years or older (approximately 75 million persons), and it was uncontrolled in roughly half of adults with hypertension (almost 35 million persons). Among these 35 million US residents with unchecked hypertension, 33 percent (11.5 million persons) are unaware of their hypertension, and 20 percent (7 million persons) are aware of their hypertension but are not treated. On the other hand, approximately 47 percent (16.1 million persons) are aware of their hypertension and are being treated for it, but treatment (by medication and lifestyle modification) is not adequately controlling their blood pressure [1].

Arterial hypertension is one of the most critical problems concerning public health globally. Its insidious development over the years makes it even more dangerous, as it does not present alarming symptoms at the outset. When they occur, hypertension is already very advanced. Hypertension is a silent assassin. Ideal blood pressure is twelve centimeters of mercury for maximum and eight centimeters for minimum pressure [2]. The continual rise in centimeters of mercury over one or two pressure readings means the tension is too high. The cardiovascular mortality rate rises immediately. Minimal tension with nine centimeters of mercury is already a bad sign. When the maximum pressure exceeds 15.8, cardiovascular risk is multiplied by 2.5. A blood pressure of 14/9 calls for immediate therapeutic measures.

The frequency of arterial hypertension is impressive. For example, Framingham, quoted by Williams and Braunwald in Harrison's *Principles of Internal Medicine* in 1989 [3], showed that in a population of white people in suburbs, 20 percent of subjects had blood pressures higher than 16/9.5, whereas 50 percent had pressures of 14/9.

These same authors specify that the cause of arterial hypertension is unknown in most cases. Doctors call this type of hypertension *essential* or *idiopathic*, meaning the etiology is unknown. Classically, it is considered a hereditary condition. Essential hypertension represents 90 percent of arterial hypertension cases.

In 2017, new guidelines from the American Heart Association, the American College of Cardiology, and nine other health organizations lowered the threshold for diagnosing hypertension to 130/80 millimeters of mercury (mm Hg) or higher for all adults. The previous guidelines set the thresholds at 140/90 mm Hg for people younger than 65 and 150/80 mm Hg for those aged 65 and older. Now, 70 to 79 percent of men aged fifty-five and older have hypertension. That includes many men whose blood pressure was previously considered healthy [4].

In April 2018, Harvard Health Publishing of the Harvard Medical School defined new blood pressure guidelines. As a result, the definition of high blood pressure has tightened. Here is what you need to know (Table 6).

Blood Pressure Categories			
Blood Pressure	Systolic mm Hg (Upper Number)		Systolic mm Hg (Lower Number)
Normal	Less than 120	and	Less than 80
Elevated	120–129	and	Less than 80
Hypertension stage 1	130–139	or	80-89
Hypertension stage 2	**140 or higher**	**or**	**90 or higher**
Hypertensive crisis	**Higher than 180**	**and**	**Higher than 120**

Table 6

The maximum and minimum arterial pressures are expressions of the variations of pressure exerted via blood on the walls of a closed elastic circuit. These pressures are caused by two engines that take turns: the cardiac muscle and the arterial musculature.

Cardiac contraction is responsible for the maximal arterial pressure, caused by the shock wave of the blood wave on the walls of large arteries, which transmit the stream in the arterial system.

The contraction of arterial muscles takes over between cardiac contractions to ensure the continuous propulsion of the blood wave through the tiny arteries (small arteries). As a result, it causes the minimum pressure. If this secondary engine did not exist, blood pressure would fall to zero between heartbeats.

Blood circulates permanently in the organs because of the successive contractions of these two powerful engines, which propel blood in the tiny arteries and the capillaries. They are the most elementary blood vessels, the last ramifications of the circulatory system, which connect small arteries and venules. This final vascular network lacks an engine; blood circulates continuously due to cardiac and arterial propulsion, which constitutes the peripheral resistance of the vascular system.

The cardiac pump must provide an extra effort to propel blood when arterial resistance increases in the large arteries: the maximum pressure rises, and heart work increases by 40 to 50 percent. The muscular pump of the arteries must also exert extra effort to propel the blood wave through the network of tiny arteries, which increases resistance; the minimum pressure thus rises.

Untreated hypertension is associated with a reduction in the life span of about ten to twenty years.

A combination of factors increases blood pressure with age. They are the rigidity of arterial walls, the increase in peripheral resistance, and the blood's high viscosity. In addition, all components must be intact for the system to work well, which is generally the case at twenty years of age.

The origin of essential hypertension is the consequence of the system's degeneration. The rigidity of arterial walls and increased peripheral resistance are the most degenerative factors.

The elasticity of arterial walls decreases because of arteriosclerosis and atheroma. These phenomena develop with age as male hormone secretion declines. It is sufficient to examine the small retinal arteries; their features are representative of those of cerebral arteries and the arterial system in general.

The increase in peripheral resistance involves a severe cardiac overload. The mass to irrigate is the resistance. How does this mass increase? The brain volume does not increase, nor does the size of other organs. What, then, can increase the human body's mass with time? Fat. It settles everywhere in the body. It is stored mainly in the belly, around the intestines of a man. One often finds there ten to twenty useless kilos. Fat is a living tissue nourished by the last ends of the arterial network, which builds up there.

Additional resistance in the arterial system increases as fatty mass increases. Because of this factor, it is necessary to act on the first extra kilo.

We saw in chapter 12 how fat tissue develops from a lack of male hormones and overeating. A blood pressure of 12/8 at 20 years of age is accompanied by a relatively low weight. If you suffer from essential hypertension, you must return to your weight at age twenty. It is entirely possible.

Hypercoagulability is also the result of the lack of male hormones. As a result, more viscous blood increases the force necessary for the propulsion of the blood wave.

Traditional hypertension treatment uses substances that affect the nervous system of muscular arteries by causing relaxation. Beta-blocker drugs, which block the action of nervous fibers that cause arterial contraction, are helpful but treat only the symptom, not the cause of hypertension. Although beta-blockers protect the heart, they cause a drop in peripheral blood pressure. For example, the arteries of the penis of a hypertensive man are part of the final network. The taking of beta-blockers makes the pressure in the penis fall, causing impotence. The same applies to the ultimate arterial system and all organs; they will suffer from a lack of irrigation.

In many cases, it is possible to be released from beta-blocker treatment by paying particular attention to weight control and decreasing arterial sclerosis with male hormones. This treatment is a correct approach from the onset of symptoms. It constitutes a significant preventive measure for hypertension. When the whole arterial system becomes rigid, it is still possible to improve the vascular state, but many lesions will become irreversible.

Hypertension causes the appearance of all kinds of mechanisms and pathological vicious circles that worsen arterial hypertension. They are responsible for many strokes and dramatic arterial ruptures.

On World Health Day 2013, the WHO published a remarkable global panorama of hypertension. It stated, "The risk of hypertension increases with age because of the hardening of the blood vessels. Although the ageing of the latter can be slowed down by adopting healthy lifestyles, including a balanced diet and a reduction in salt consumption."

Certain people limit their blood pressure by changing their lifestyles, for example, stopping tobacco use, eating healthily, getting regular physical exercise, and avoiding the harmful use of alcohol. However, all adults should control their blood pressure. If it rises, they must consult a health professional.

The lack of testosterone responsible for arteriosclerosis is the leading cause of essential arterial hypertension in men who need individual attention. Mesterolone is the proper treatment for technical reasons, not testosterone (see chapter 33).

Fibrous tissue replaces arterial muscle and degenerating fibers. But, at first visible only at the microscopic level, fibrosis constitutes a dynamic obstacle to blood flow in the absence of arterial narrowing visible to the eye (chapter 14).

Variations in Blood pressure, in Centimeters of Mercury According to Age, in 250,000 Americans in Good Health		
Age	Maximum pressure	Minimum pressure
10	10.3	7
15	11.3	7.5
20	12	8
25	12.2	8.1
30	12.3	8.2
35	12.4	8.3
40	12.6	8.4
45	12.8	8.5
50	13	8.6
55	13.2	8.7
60	13.5	8.9

Table 7

Statistics of Hunter quoted by Best and Taylor [2].

Essential hypertension represents 90 percent of arterial hypertension cases resulting from arteriosclerosis. The cause of arteriosclerosis is the progressive atrophy of arterial muscle fibers due to a lack of anabolic hormones from age twenty-five.

The blood pressure of 12/8 is normal. It is the case at age twenty.

Table 15 shows the progressive elevation of blood pressure after age twenty. Remarkably, blood pressure had already increased moderately at twenty-five. However, the maximum and minimum pressures increase continually from age twenty-five to sixty.

Hypertension intensifies with age across the whole population [2], which raises the question of a fundamental cause that accentuates its effects over time.

At age twenty-five, the human being is in top form, with average quantities of anabolic hormones produced by the body. However, from age twenty-five on, the production of male hormones decreases in parallel with increased blood pressure. This phenomenon is the cause of arteriosclerosis.

Coronary Disease and Heart Infarct

Cardiac Diseases and Atheroma

Angina pectoris is the expression of a temporary reduction in the oxygenation of the cardiac muscle.

The work of the heart requires a continuous supply of oxygen, transported by blood that circulates through the coronary arteries. There are two. One irrigates the front wall of the heart; the other, the back wall. These two arteries meet in the cardiac muscle.

The most frequent cause of angina pectoris in a man with an androgenic disease of andropause is atherosclerosis of the coronary arteries. It is made up of fatty deposits that decrease the diameter of the principal or secondary arteries in one or more places.

Emotional factors can also trigger an angina pectoris crisis by producing an intense spasm of the heart's arteries, leading to insufficient irrigation of the cardiac muscle.

The contribution of oxygenated blood decreases more significantly as the arteries are narrowed. In the beginning, reduced physical activity does not start the crisis. The insufficiency of blood irrigation appears during a physical effort, which causes precordial pain. The contribution of the blood cannot ensure sufficient oxygenation of the heart during this extra work. The crisis occurs, for example, while running to catch the train or the bus.

Arterial flow is insufficient at rest when the arterial diameter is reduced by more than 80%. Crises occur at any time, even in bed.

More arterial gauge reduction causes dramatic heart diseases like myocardial infarction. In addition, a tight constriction of the anterior coronary artery causes a mortality rate of 15 percent yearly.

Electrocardiograms show characteristic signs when heart artery contraction is problematic. At rest, these modifications are not always manifest if the arteries are moderately narrowed. In this case, electrocardiographic changes are demonstrated by a stress test. The electrocardiogram is recorded during the bicycle stress test under the cardiologist's supervision.

The localization of the arterial narrowing is demonstrated by coronary angiography (heart artery radiographs). A catheter, introduced into a large leg artery, is advanced toward the heart and selectively navigated into the coronary artery to inject a contrast medium.

Cardiovascular mortality correlates with the evolution of atheroma deposits in the heart's arteries. The rise in blood fats (triglycerides) significantly increases the risk of narrowing the heart arteries. Likewise, the increase in "bad" cholesterol (low-density lipoprotein [LDL] cholesterol) is in correlation with coronary insufficiency.

Studies have shown the crucial role of "good" cholesterol (high-density lipoprotein [HDL]) in preventing coronary disease. Cholesterol is transported in the blood by specific proteins. Its principal function is to collect cholesterol in several sites and carry it toward the liver, where it is degraded and excreted in the bile. HDL proteins are, all in all, the "street sweepers" of cholesterol.

The Framingham Heart Study showed that, for both men and women, an HDL cholesterol level above 52 milligrams per hundred cubic centimeters of plasma is a protective factor against the risk of coronary insufficiency [1].

Foods rich in animal fats raise harmful blood fats and contribute to the development of cardiovascular disease.

On the other hand, populations that stick to a vegetarian diet low in fats are less predisposed to cardiovascular diseases. The Bantu vegetarians, for example, experienced a rise in blood cholesterol after leaving the rural areas for the city and modifying their dietary habits by eating Western food.

A man with coronary insufficiency must reexamine his lifestyle by controlling his food intake and physical activity. In addition, he must avoid smoking and eliminate any causes of stress.

High level	Correlation with coronary insufficiency
Total cholesterol	+
LDL cholesterol	+
Triglycerides	+
HDL cholesterol	-

Table 8

Testosterone Deficit and Cardiac Diseases

Deficits in male hormones and disturbances in their metabolism have been correlated with cardiac disease for about fifty years, and the first treatments with testosterone date back to that time.

Coronary Insufficiency

Angina pectoris is a transitory pain felt at the level of the heart. Men account for 80 percent of cases beyond age fifty and a higher percentage before this age. The pain is a discomfort in the chest, where it appears. There is a heaviness, a feeling of oppression or smothering, or an impression of squeezing or compression. The intensity of this discomfort is generally variable and lasts 1 to 5 minutes. The pain can be perceived in the left shoulder and the arms.

The narrowing of the coronary arteries correlates with disturbances in sex hormone levels. This lesser-known reality, however, is essential. Coronary insufficiency is associated with the disorder of sex hormone levels in men. Male hormones, testosterone, and dihydrotestosterone are in perpetual balance with the female hormone estradiol in men.

The heart functions well when male hormones are raised, and female hormones do not exceed the ideal level of twenty picograms per milliliter of plasma (radioimmunology analysis). An excess of female hormones neutralizes male hormones.

Several studies showed the correlation between coronary insufficiency and the existence, on the one hand, of a low testosterone level and, on the other hand, of a high female hormone level. The proportions of male and female hormones can be simultaneously disturbed. An insufficient level of dihydrotestosterone is also correlated with coronary insufficiency (Table 9).

The traditional treatment of coronary insufficiency does not consider the crucial role of male hormones. However, individual doctors have understood it and successfully treated heart cases with male hormones.

In 1946, Lesser published a study on 101 patients suffering from angina pectoris, treated with testosterone propionate [2]. There were ninety-two men and eight women, ranging from thirty-four to seventy-seven years old. The average treatment was carried out with 12 intramuscular injections.

A reference group of patients receiving sesame oil injections not containing hormones showed no improvement in the painful symptoms. However, these patients, treated with testosterone, reacted favorably to the treatment and did not show any undesirable effects.

Hormone	Plasma level	Correlation with coronary insufficiency
Total testosterone	Low	+
Free testosterone	Low	+
Dihydrotestosterone	Low	+
Estradiol	Raised	+

Table 9

Four patients were given stress tests before and during the hormonal therapy to measure the improvement of their cardiac states objectively. As a result, each of them could expend more effort during the hormonal treatment than in their former conditions, and the duration of painful heart attacks was shortened. In each case, subjective improvement preceded objective measurements of improved cardiac work.

Jens Møeller, in Copenhagen, prescribed male hormones for more than thirty years to treat cardiovascular diseases. In 1984, he published his experience in a book, *Testosterone Treatment of Cardiovascular Diseases* [3]. In 1987, Møeller again covered the same topic in a second work, *Cholesterol* [4], and concluded that testosterone plays a crucial role in treating cardiovascular diseases. According to this author, the delay in combating these diseases with hormonal therapy is due to the inability of many specialists in endocrinology, biochemistry, physiology, and cardiology to understand one another's points of view. Møeller compares this phenomenon to a pyramid, with each face climbed by a person who does not see the others before reaching the top.

An insufficiency of the secretion of male sex hormones intervenes decisively in a disordered state of metabolism of sugars, fats, and cholesterol. This lack is responsible for arteriosclerosis and atheroma. The correlation between hormonal insufficiency and coronary insufficiency is well established.

Heart Infarct

Until the eighteenth century, cardiac diseases were unknown and even denied. Diderot affirms in his *Encyclopedia* that heart diseases were uncommon.

During the twentieth century, especially after 1940, heart diseases became the focus of attention, coronary syndromes constituting a disaster in industrialized countries.

When the arteries of the heart are narrowed, blood supply to certain parts of the cardiac muscle is reduced, leading to necrosis, sometimes dramatically.

The heart was, from time immemorial, regarded as the center of the human. It became the emblem of courage, intelligence, and friendship. In a word, the heart symbolizes love. More prosaically, the heart is an automatic muscle, but before all, a muscle. To contract, it needs, like the skeletal muscle, the force of contractile proteins and fuel—glycogen, which is fundamental.

The chemistry of cardiac muscle contraction depends on the action of male hormones. They are specific receptors for testosterone in the muscle fibers of a rat's heart [5,6]. Other experiments have shown increased actinomyosin content in cardiac muscle with testosterone administration [7]. This substance reinforces the specific contractile elements.

Older heart disease sufferers have been advised to take all kinds of drugs for their heart problems. But do they know that an essential "food" for the heart, testosterone, is missing? Male hormones reinforce the muscular contraction of cardiac muscle, just as they reinforce the actions of the other muscular tissues. Taking androgens improves the work of the insufficient or degenerated heart.

In 1996, Dominique Simon (of unit 21 of the INSERM [the French National Institute of Health and Medical Research]), Khalil Nahoul, and their collaborators confirmed the favorable impact of testosterone on cardiovascular risk factors. This study, known as the Telecom Study [8], spanned 8 years and compared cardiovascular risk parameters between two groups (HDL cholesterol, LDL cholesterol, triglycerides, blood sugar, and so on).

The first group, whose blood testosterone levels remained stable for eight years, showed no increase in vascular risk for this period. However, the second group, whose blood testosterone levels decreased for this period, showed a significant increase in cardiovascular risk [8].

Androgen hormones, when well-proportioned, naturally decrease cholesterol levels. In this case, one can observe a decrease in good cholesterol (HDL cholesterol) in the blood. In 2012, a study by the University of Washington School of Medicine in Seattle showed that this reduction corresponds to accelerated HDL cholesterol transport [9].

In the same year, researchers in the Cardiovascular Department of Medicine at the University of Harbin in China reported an exciting finding in castrated rats. Those animals had a heart infarct following the binding of a coronary artery. In addition, testosterone replacement therapy led to the formation of new blood vessels [10].

Myocardial infarction is the final expression of a morbid process generated by the lack of energy substances necessary to the cardiac muscle, worsened by degeneration of the coronary arteries.

Male hormones thin the blood and increase the contractile force of the cardiac muscle. As a result, they support healing by stimulating protein synthesis and causing heart revascularization.

19

Stiffnesses, Limitation of Movement, Slipped Discs, and Degenerative Joint Disease

Stiffness moves with age. The penis becomes increasingly soft while the ligaments, the tendons, and the fibrous tissue of the organism retract. We know that organic impotence, which appears with age, is the consequence of reduced secretion of male hormones. One can wonder whether the same cause is not responsible for stiffness and limited movement. At first sight, we do not see the relationship. The idea could even appear fanciful.

Causes of Degenerative Joint Disease

Knowing some elements of the nature and biochemistry of conjunctive tissues is necessary. These tissues occupy the intervals between the organs and constitute the details of an organ. They are components of mechanical support and framing. They consist of cells and fibers that "bathe" in a kind of gel (fundamental substance) made up of specialized molecules. Through the conjunctive tissue, nutritive molecules and oxygen arrive in the organism's cells.

Fibrocytes, the conjunctive cells, generate fibers. The most well-known are collagenous fibers. They meet in almost all conjunctive tissues and consist of subunits outside the cells that formed them. The *collagenous* (in French, from *colle* and *gene*) qualifier comes from the name of the proteins that constitute these fibers. They are transformed into gelatin by heat.

The high resistance of collagen to traction confers the solidity of conjunctive tissues.

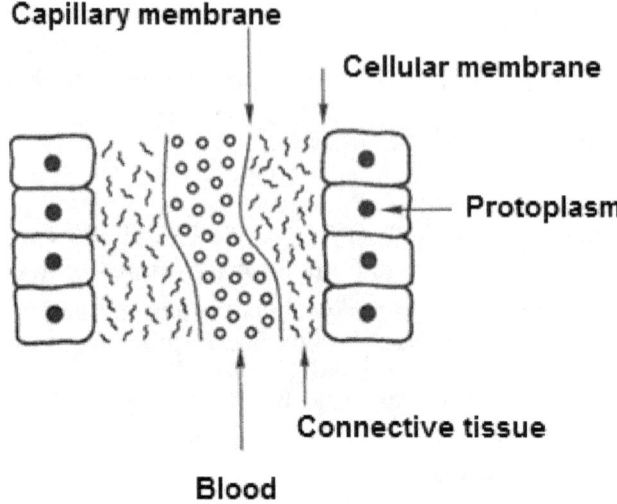

Fig. 17

Diagram of the barrier between blood and tissues, After Sobel and Marmorston [4]

The tangle of fibers adapts perfectly to the structures that surround specific tissues. Collagenous fibers constitute the essence of ligament and tendon structures, perhaps the best known being the Achilles tendon. Inserted in the heel's bone, it is prone to injuries and ruptures during excessive physical effort.

Collagenous proteins have a probable lifespan of several years, but measuring them is difficult. In the event of wounds, specialized cells make new fibers to fill the gap, constituting scar tissue.

Ligaments and tendons retract with age. Pick up a paper from the ground, or putting on a coat becomes an increasingly complex operation.

Thus, the cells of the organism age, but the matter that surrounds and supports them ages as well. This phenomenon was demonstrated in the famous experiments of the Hungarian physiologist Fritz Verzar. He suspended collagen filaments from a rat's tail in a bain-marie at a temperature of thirty-seven to forty degrees. Under these conditions, the fibers shortened, and collagen proteins denatured in gelatin.

One can prevent the shortening by suspending a weight at the end of the fibers. The load required to prevent shortening is more significant in older animals [1,2].

As we age, collagen becomes more resistant rather than weakening because the elementary collagen fibers are connected to one another by chemical bridges. Increased resistance and retraction of collagen with age are consequences of increased numbers of bridges or changes in their chemical nature.

Glucose binds to all proteins. The excessive presence of glucose in the body accentuates the structural transformation of healthy collagen into a rigid form. The billions of glucose molecules "stick" chemically to the elementary collagen fibers between them [3]. All conditions that abnormally raise blood glucose cause the abnormal bridging of collagen. Male hormones play a crucial role in lowering blood glucose levels (chapter 10).

Insufficient secretion of male hormones leads to a tendency toward increased blood sugar, which, in turn, is responsible for abnormal collagen bridging, leading to retraction of ligaments and tendons. For this reason, while being "too sweetened," the man with an androgenic disease of andropause becomes stiff.

Rigid collagenous fibers and cells bathe in a gelatinous substance. This gel is a required mechanism for transporting nutritive molecules and oxygen within cells. However, with age, the composition of this extracellular gel deteriorates, compromising the nutrition of cellular compartments.

The scarcity of the gelatinous substance is a consequence of the insufficiency of the secretion of male hormones. This phenomenon was shown in 1958 by Sobel and Marmorston from the Institute for Medical Research, Cedars of Lebanon Hospital, and the Department of Biochemistry and Nutrition and the Department of Medicine, University of Southern California, Los Angeles, California [4].

Hand Pains

Fibrosis and retraction of the wrist's ligaments can compress the nerves that arrive at the hand. Under these conditions, the median nerve can be compressed, causing pain in the thumb, index, or middle finger. Specialized surgery that decompresses nerves eliminates the pain.

Finger Retractions

Retraction of the superficial fascia, which covers the palm, is spectacular. It is the Dupuytren disease. The fingers curl up and become immobilized in this position. To correct this infirmity, traditional treatment resorts to specialized surgery that treats the consequences of the disease rather than its cause. The operation does not prevent repetition.

Retraction of the hand's ligaments depends on hormonal balance, which modifies the fibrous tissue's composition and causes contraction of the tiny arteries. Therefore, it is always necessary to act from the beginning of the disease, correcting what it might lead to without waiting for curled fingers. A lack of male hormones triggers a series of biochemical reactions that lead to the degeneration and retraction of tendons and ligaments.

Dupuytren's disease is an age-related disease. Classically, its cause is not of androgens indicate insufficient production of androgens. Mesterolone, from the first known. In our experience, it is caused in men and women when low levels symptoms, prevents the disease from progressing and avoids the need for surgery [5]. However, further research will be needed in this field.

Slipped Discs

Vertebrae are separated by intervertebral discs, which cushion the impact of shocks on the vertebrae. The intervertebral disc degenerates due to a lack of male hormones and becomes thin. The overlying and underlying vertebrae move toward each other, causing a vertebral "pinching" at the origin of often intolerable pain caused by excessive pressure on the nerves that leave the spinal column. This widespread phenomenon in men with an androgenic andropause disease usually requires surgery to decompress the crushed nerves. The supervening of a first slipped disc in a man with the androgenic illness of andropause is a severe symptom. This degeneration signals further degeneration of his joint articulations and ligaments. Then, the totality of his body degenerates due to a lack of male hormones that have the biological property of rebuilding intervertebral ligaments, discs, and articulations.

When male hormone secretion is insufficient, slipped disc recurrence is the rule, leading to new surgeries.

The joint articulations degenerate on one side or both sides. Being overweight worsens the excessive pressure on afflicted articulations, thus delaying the healing of any surgical procedure.

The slimming decreases muscular force, regardless of the regime, leading to a functional overload of the affected and operated-on articulations. The slimming diet will have better results by administering male hormones, decreasing fat, and improving mass and muscular force (see chapters 12 and 13).

The situation is further complicated by infection of surgically treated articulations. Because in a man with the androgenic disease of andropause, his immune system can be defective (see chapter 26).

Cascading catastrophes lead to multiple surgical procedures, which could be avoided by preventing degeneration with male hormones.

The biological rebuilding of discs, ligaments, and articulations could take several years when hormonal treatment was ignored and replaced by successive surgical procedures. Hormonal therapy can be lifesaving.

Degenerative Joint Disease or Osteoarthritis

Osteoarthritis is a degenerative disease of the joint articulations. All are involved, but those used for support are particularly predisposed.

Osteoarthritis is common in men after age forty-five and becomes more common with age. However, it is practically constant after age seventy-five.

Movement confers on men their physical freedom and autonomy, which are essential to survival. Mobility characterizes a particular functional entity: articulation. The cartilage facilitates support and slip functions, covering the two osseous ends linked by a capsule and ligaments. The joint capsule is lined inside by a specialized synovial membrane that produces a lubricating fluid, synovial fluid. Muscles inserted on both sides of the osseous ends constitute the engine of articulation.

This functional entity is nourished by an arterial network, which ends in small arteries.

In the beginning, osteoarthritis appears as a limitation of movements. Pain clears up in the morning and disappears during the day. At this stage, the articulation does not show a clinical sign. Gradually, the motion becomes more limited due to ligament retraction and rigidity, which form calcium deposits and produce crackling noises. While turning the head, for example, one perceives small cracklings in the neck.

This stage is already significant. It is here that it is necessary to act quickly. The diagnosis is based primarily on normal radiographs. Only bones are visible on radiographs of the four articular structures—the bone, the synovial membrane, the joint capsule, and the cartilage. The other structures are radiotransparent. Moreover, one needs to understand the essential variation in its calcium load to appreciate a modification in the skeletal structure. When calcium loss reaches approximately 30 percent, one can detect an osseous decalcification with radiographs.

After many months and many years, the diagnosis of osteoarthritis finally becomes visible on radiographs. Articulation degeneration appears through cartilage destruction and the approach of the bony end. One feels articular pinching. The calcified ligaments and the joint capsule are visible around the articulation. Finally, overloaded with calcium, the ends of the bones are sometimes welded together, immobilizing the bones. Everyone knows a grandmother or grandfather with osteoarthritis. It usually began at age forty and was never cured. Nothing is currently done to prevent this degenerative phenomenon that ultimately strikes all older men.

All articulations undergo the same fate. The degenerative aspects are marked in the knee, hip, spinal column, and shoulder, which work more.

Knee osteoarthritis presents with pain when going up and down stairs. The knee inflates, and the kneecap immobilizes. One can remove the joint surgically and replace it with an artificial knee when joint articulation is blocked. Knee osteoarthritis is an important topic because it affects the quality of life of millions of people.

The prevalence of hip osteoarthritis is higher among men younger than fifty, whereas women have the highest incidence after age fifty because of postmenopausal changes. It strikes both hips in 20 percent of cases. Pain while walking is perceived in the groin, buttocks, thighs, and the knee, and calms at rest. The articulation worsens gradually. The head of the femur, formerly round, is flattened into the shape of a "coach buffer." The bony cavity in which it is encased is overloaded with calcium and develops excrescences, immobilizing the articulation completely. The gait becomes lame. It is challenging to rise from a seated position—consequently, the muscles surrounding the articulation degenerate, producing a trailing gait.

That is no problem, traditional medicine will say; surgery is there to remove the affected articulation and replace it with a prosthesis. Unfortunately, the results are not definitive because the bone around the prosthesis worsens again. Many men undergo multiple replacements of hip prostheses, increasing the number of complicated and hazardous surgical procedures.

Vertebral osteoarthritis involves the cervical, dorsal, or lumbar segments of the spinal column. One notes the calcareous overload of ligaments and osseous excrescences ("parrots' nozzles"). The vertebrae's collapse can pinch the nerves that leave the spinal column, sometimes causing intolerable pain. That is no problem either; traditional medicine might say surgery is there to decompress the wedged nerve. But surgery is not definitive. The bony substance worsens again, leading to recurrence at the operated site or above or below it.

The cervical and lumbar columns are reached first for mechanical reasons.

Osteoarthritis of the cervical column causes pain in the nape, sometimes radiating to the arm.

Compression of specific nerve roots causes headaches, giddiness, eye or ear problems, and pain. In addition, neck mobilization is limited, resulting in crackling.

Osteoarthritis of the dorsal column is rarer. Nerve pinching causes intercostal pain.

Lumbar osteoarthritis is widespread. At first, after a little physical effort, it appears that a severe lumbago crisis is developing. The spasm of lumbar muscles immobilizes the patient for a few hours to a few days. This benign incident recurs.

Pain also radiates to the thighs and buttocks and the testicles in men. Sciatic nerve compression is particularly painful. It begins in the lumbar area, is propagated in the outer face of the leg, and finishes in the big toe. At an advanced stage, pain becomes permanent and prevents even the slightest movement.

Many causes of osteoarthritis are known. They all lead to the destruction of the cartilage, the true shock absorber of the joint. With time, the cartilage wears out like the car's shock absorbers.

Generally, the causes reside, on the one hand, in mechanical disorders of articulation (poorly assembled shock absorbers or having received an excessive shock) and, on the other hand, in structural conditions of the articulation itself (shock absorbers of poor quality).

Ageing contributes to the development of hip osteoarthritis, mainly because of the inability to correctly define an underlying anatomic abnormality or specific disease process leading to the degenerative process. Osteoarthritis of unknown origin accounts for 50 percent of the cases, gradually destroying the whole articular system. Medical books describe *primitive osteoarthritis* as a term for osteoarthritis of unknown origin, which means nothing for prevention and treatment.

One can wonder about a general cause that worsens with age.

The traditional treatment of osteoarthritis of unknown origin is primarily symptomatic and relates to its consequences. Pain can be relieved by aspirin. Anti-inflammatory drugs are not without disadvantages. They can cause bleeding or disorders of blood composition. Doctors sometimes inject cortisone into or around the joint to reduce inflammation. These infiltrations must be made judiciously and not repeated too often.

Failure of these treatments leads to osteopathy or manual therapy, which temporarily relieves the patient's symptoms. Lastly, surgery promptly replaces the completely worn joints when other options have failed.

Treatment of Degenerative Joint Disease with Male Hormones

During hormonal treatments for sexual insufficiency, my attention was often drawn to the reflections of patients who announced to me the disappearance of their shoulder, knee, or finger pain. "It is strange; my pains disappeared," they said.

At first, I did not attach importance to these comments. Then, however, the repetition of these surprising testimonies convinced me that male hormones act on osteoarthritis and prevent its development independently of any other factor. While reflecting, I realized that this fact is not astonishing for two reasons.

The first reason concerns the vascularization of the articulations. They are tiny arteries, without which neither oxygen nor nutritive substances can arrive at the specialized cells.

The cartilage does not contain small arteries; it is nourished by imbibition, starting from the articular liquid secreted by the synovial membrane, or diffusion, beginning from the end of the bone where they branch, ending with the smallest arteries.

The small arteries degenerate when arteriosclerosis develops. We observed that arteriosclerosis develops more rapidly when male hormones are deficient. Consequently, the secretion of the articular fluid will be compromised.

The second reason concerns cartilage, mainly consisting of a fundamental substance that confers elasticity and resistance to an organism. One also finds collagenous fibers. Specialized cells in cartilage produce these protein structures. They constitute a living tissue that requires continuous maintenance. When male hormones are insufficient, protein synthesis is compromised, leading to cartilage degeneration.

These two essential consequences of the lack of male hormones seriously compromise the structures of all articulations. Osteoarthritis worsens even more in a man with excess weight.

Many cases of osteoarthritis of unknown origin result from arteriosclerosis of the tiny joint arteries. At the same time, the insufficiency of male hormone secretion provokes the degeneration of the articular cartilage. Preventing osteoarthritis in time with mesterolone, in combination with diet, is a possible solution. When destroyed, however, articulations need conventional treatment.

Fragile Bones

We see many falls and blows to the tibiae during football matches. Sometimes, their violence is so considerable that one can fear osseous fractures, nailing players on the ground. Nothing comes of it. They rise and invariably play again. The age of footballers oscillates. For the majority, for around twenty-five years, their bones are solid.

The other day, a doctor, fifty-five years old, came to consult me for initial sexual disorders. He knew the importance of sex hormones in this field and thought of needing treatment. All his clinical history demonstrated an insufficiency of male hormone secretion. I prescribed hormonal analyses, thinking of reexamining him a few days later. While returning home, he slipped inopportunely, making a simple fall. Impossible for him to get up; he was transported to the hospital with a hip fracture. Hormonal analyses showed a manifest insufficiency of male hormones.

Thirty years separate our young, impetuous footballers from this unhappy man—thirty critical years. Yet, simple good sense makes it possible to bring the two cases closer: young and healthy players, entirely impregnated by abundant secretion of male hormones, and an out-of-date and fragile man deprived of them.

Like all support tissues, bone tissue consists of specialized cells, fibers, and a fundamental substance. The bones accumulate mineral salts, especially calcium salts, which give them rigidity and consistency.

Bone tissue has mechanical functions of support or protection. The pressure resistance of compact bone tissue is fifteen kilos per square millimeter. Moreover, the bone resists inflection and presents a certain degree of elasticity.

The bone is also a chemical tank. Its structural makeup continuously modifies the distribution of mineral salts. Chemical reserves of bones produce a renewal of calcium and phosphorus. Contrary to cartilage, tiny arteries irrigate the bones.

The skeletal structure is also influenced by male hormones. The maturation of the skeleton during adolescence testifies to its fundamental impact. It is well established that a defect of male hormones induces a slenderness ratio of the bones and that excellent hormonal secretion gives a robust skeletal constitution. Conversely, when growing old, the bone structure weakens for four fundamental reasons caused by a lack of male hormones:

• Bone vascularization consists of a network of narrow arteries reaching osseous ends. They take part in generalized arteriosclerosis. The consequence is poor oxygenation of the articulations.

• Skeletal structures break up gradually. The collagenous fibers and the fundamental substance* participate in the degradation that affects all protein structures in the organism.

• Calcium is poorly fixed on support tissue, causing bone porosity.

• Rarefaction of bone tissue is called *osteoporosis*. The bone is the seat of permanent remodeling. Its integrity depends on the balance between destruction and construction in the skeletal substance. Cortisol secreted by the suprarenal glands accentuates the process of decay. The structure of the skeleton depends on testosterone. At the time of andropause, cortisol's effects exceed testosterone's constructive properties, and osteoporosis develops.

In men, the osseous loss is accentuated with age and the lack of testosterone. There is a linear relationship between the plasma

---

* The collagenous fibers and the fundamental substance consist of proteins (see chapter 19).

testosterone level and bone density. The diagnosis of osseous brittleness is made on radiographs, which invariably show bone transparency, evidence of brittleness. One needs a calcium deficit of approximately 30% to detect bone decalcification on X-rays. Thus, the radiological diagnosis is too late. Today, a more precise method of examining bone density, quantitative computed tomography, is available, enabling early diagnosis of osteoporosis and facilitating tracking of its regression with male hormone treatment.

Years of rheumatism and joint pain precede osteoporosis. Over time, bone tissue is packed, and a man with an androgenic disease of andropause may lose several centimeters in height. His bones become fragile, like glass. A minor fall results in fractures. Lack of male hormones causes osseous brittleness in men with an androgenic disease of andropause.

The teeth are implanted in the bone and held in place by ligaments. These structures degenerate, as does the body's structure when testosterone is lacking. Tooth loosening is worsened by poor dental hygiene and excessive sugar intake, leading to gum detachment and the formation of purulent pockets around dental roots.

A study on ageing was published in 2013 by the Geriatric Research Center of the University of Changsha, Hunan, China. This clinical research was conducted on men with osteoporosis and low plasma testosterone. It showed the beneficial effects of small amounts of testosterone undecanoate on osseous mineral density [1].

21

Skin Wrinkles

The skin plays a significant role in the organism. In the adult male, its weight can range from 13 to 22 pounds for a surface area of 1.6 square meters. The skin can be observed in depth without difficulty, and the modifications caused by age are visible as soon as they appear after age forty-five.

The cutaneous coating is a structure composed of various elements. The epidermis is the outer layer of the two layers that make up the skin, the inner layer being the dermis.

The epidermis consists of superimposed cell layers; the deepest are flexible. The superficial cells constitute the cornified layer—these separate from the deep layer due to burning (sunburn), forming blisters. In a healthy state, cornified cells flake off as a powder.

The central part of the skin, the dermis, contains many elastic fibers that serve as cutaneous tensioners, responsible for smooth skin. In addition, deep dermis cells produce a grease that constitutes a protective coating against the cold.

The skin contains two significant types of glands, those that secrete grease (sebaceous glands) and others that secrete sweat (sudoriferous glands).

The sebaceous glands are in the deep part of the skin and are generally attached to hairs. Relatively rare on the chest, the neck, and the palms and soles, they are, on the contrary, numerous in certain areas, such as the scalp and the nose; there, one finds four hundred glands or more per square centimeter of human skin.

In the deep part of the skin, they are sudoriferous glands. There are approximately two hundred sudoriferous glands per square centimeter of skin, and their total number is three million for the whole of the cutaneous coating. The system of sudoriferous organs secretes about one liter of sweat per day; it can provide five to six liters or more.

The skin protects the organism from shocks and chemical aggression. It plays a significant role in thermal regulation, breathing, and elimination of the organism's waste (e.g., urea, rock salts). Extremely rich in nervous terminations, the skin is an organ of sensitivity and reflectivity. The skin and its annexes are large consumers of male hormones. Old skin is characteristic of a man with androgen deficiency (andropause). Degenerative demonstrations are multiple. They are visible to the naked eye and draw attention, but their effects can be mitigated with appropriate hormonal treatment. With age, the superficial part of the skin thins. There are atrophied zones and young skin. With advanced age, the skin becomes extremely fine, particularly on the back of the hands and the legs. In old age, the skin becomes as thin as cigarette paper. It is also poorly irrigated, bloodless, and pale.

Young skin is elastic; old skin is not. Cutaneous elasticity results from the quality of collagenous fibers, elastic fibers, and dermal muscles* With age, collagenous tissues become rigid, and elastic fibers lose their elasticity. The phenomenon usually begins around age forty-five, but can occur as early as age thirty-five.

With time, the skin of the thorax tends to slip; the inner sides of the arms float when one raises them horizontally; and the inner parts of the thighs float like a flag.

The dermal muscles take part in the generalized muscular atrophy of andropause. There are muscles in the eyelids, the lips, the cheeks, the face, and the neck. All the muscles of mimicry are atrophied gradually

---

* The dermal muscles are superficial and insert into the deep dermis.

by a lack of male hormones. The folded skin tends to hang. Drooping upper eyelids produce slanting eyes.

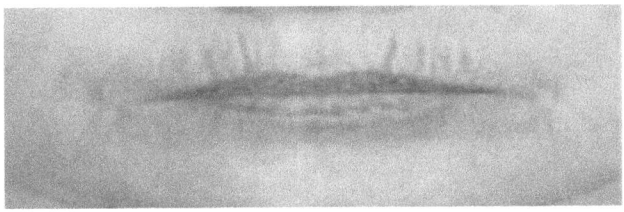

Fig. 18

Lip wrinkles.

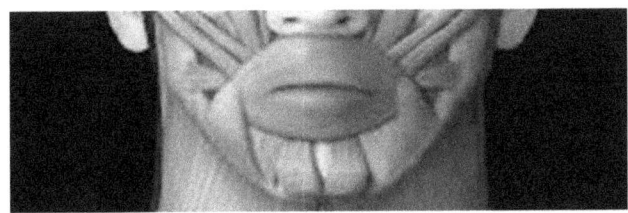

Fig. 19

Normal lip musculature.

The drooping lower lip gives projects the impression of a sulky person. The upper lip narrows and presents many vertical wrinkles (figure 18).

Drooping cheeks result in jowls along the jaw. The face has vertical creases above the nose root and a succession of horizontal lines. The neck is folded. The lifelessness of the dermal muscles accentuates expression wrinkles, which deepen further due to muscular weakness. This reality can be masked when the face is invaded by fat, appearing as joviality (one may fear that losing weight will cause wrinkles). The look of an untreated man is marked by unhappiness or false air.

Injection of a collagenous substance into wrinkles is popular today. The result is only temporary. Treatment with mesterolone maintains the elastic qualities of the skin and the lip muscles; it constitutes a natural, permanent biochemical muscular facelift.

Sweat production drops dramatically after approximately age 60 because the skin's water supply is compromised. As a result, the skin is always dry, making it impossible to sweat. Consequently, heat intolerance is accompanied by a fine exfoliative powder of dead cells. In addition, there is a reduction in sebum secretion* by the sebaceous glands [1].

Skin that renews too slowly is poorly irrigated and scarcely defended against infection. The most common is the consequence of colonization by a fungal organism, *Candida albicans*. It develops between the toes, within the circumference of the nails in the feet and fingers, the cutaneous folds, the foreskin, and the scrotum. Itching and burning follow, requiring antifungal treatment.

The skin contains specialized cells (melanocytes) that produce the pigment melanin, which is responsible for skin tanning. Melanin protects the skin from solar radiation. The skin browns more, especially when melanocyte activity is high. The ageing of the skin is characterized by excessive, localized accumulations of melanin pigment. Brown spots make their appearance on the back of the hands, the forearms, the face, and the scalp. They are of variable size and form. They are commonly called "flowers of the cemetery."

---

* Sebum is a smooth fat. It contains protein substances and is produced by sebaceous glands and the waste of secreting cells.

The skin produces less melanin pigment in a man with androgen deficiency (andropause). As a result, it reddens but does not brown, making exposure to the sun unbearable.

The skin of older men is also prone to small, spontaneous bleeds due to the relaxation of cutaneous support tissue. In addition, the protection of the small, fragile dermal vessels is not assured; their walls tear with minor stretching or trauma. Healing of these lesions causes star-shaped white scars.

Phimosis

In men with phimosis, the foreskin* covers the glans penis permanently, even in an erect state. Like the whole genitals, the foreskin is particularly sensitive to male hormones. In their absence, the skin that covers the glans penis atrophies. It becomes rigid and is easily infected. With time, the foreskin forms a sclerosed ring in front of the glans penis, which cannot be discovered anymore. This abnormal narrowness of the foreskin is called phimosis. In the best cases, the foreskin becomes flexible after disinfection and with the local application of a cream containing male hormones. When the ring remains rigid despite the hormonal treatment, one can consider the correction of the sick foreskin with benign surgery done carefully through an anatomical reconstruction†.

Hair and nails constitute the appendages of the skin. Hair grows back after a long time. Although the eyelashes of eyelids have only a short life, the hairs can persist from three to five years. New hairs replace them after their loss. Hair grows at a rate of 0.2 to 0.4 millimeters per

---

* The fold of skin that covers the penis glans.

† The anatomical reconstruction of the foreskin is limited in correcting its anomalies. The sclerosed ring is eliminated, without resorting to the traditional circumcision, which eliminates most of the foreskin and its innervation.

day. Hair lengthens 1.5 millimeters per week on the leg, and those of the pubis and the armpits, 2.2 millimeters.

With age, hair tends to become sparse on the arms, legs, chest, armpits, and pubis because its growth depends on male hormones. Hair bleaches from a lack of melanin pigment. Hair growth relies on the activity of the thyroid gland, whose insufficiency can be suspected when hair loss is abnormal.

Nails are corneous plates that protect the ends of the fingers and toes. They consist of a protein, keratin. Usually, the nails must be hard. Their growth is practically indefinite. In men, development is more active between the ages of 5 and 30. Growth ranges from approximately one millimeter per week for the fingernails to 0.25 millimeters for toenails. The nails become thin, cracked, and prone to breaking when male hormones are lacking. As a result, they no longer grow and become sites of fungal infections.

22

Shortness of Breath

With age, it is not so easy to extinguish all the candles on the birthday cake by blowing only once, especially when they are numerous. Nevertheless, the test is familiar, and one is delighted when their grandfather succeeds after several times because it is, for him, a sign of great vitality.

The gaseous exchange between blood and the air depends primarily on the lung, which resembles a considerable sponge full of air. The cavities of this sponge consist of cells with small walls. Capillaries irrigate each cell, whose walls are thin*.

The cells are supported by tiny conjunctive tissues that ensure a certain lung elasticity. Inhalation depends on the respiratory muscles, which cause the expansion of the lungs. During exhalation, a passive phenomenon, the lung returns due to the cells' elastic formations. The maximum quantity of air expelled after a full inhalation is 3.8 liters.

Chronic pulmonary emphysema is a permanent dilation of the air cells and the small bronchi. The capacity of lung ventilation is reduced, leading to poor air renewal. The thorax takes the barrel shape, and the neck seems too short. The respiratory movements are limited or even absent. The breath is missing. Speaking is also challenging. The oxygen–blood transfer surface is reduced, creating extra work for the heart.

---

* The entire surface of the alveolar walls is estimated at ninety square meters in men, and the maximum surface of the opened capillary network is 140 square meters. The gaseous exchange is made only by the diffusion between the air and the content of gas in the blood.

The principal mechanism of emphysema caused by ageing is a loss of elasticity of the lung's connective tissue. During exhalation, the lung cannot retract entirely. The generalised ageing of conjunctive tissue acts at the pulmonary level. See the discussion of the mechanism of this degeneration in chapter 19.

Senile emphysema is worsened by tobacco use, which provokes complex chemical reactions and destroys pulmonary elastic tissue.

The traditional treatment of emphysema includes bronchial drainage, bronchodilator drugs, antibiotics, and respiratory rehabilitation. But, as always, this treatment bears on the consequences of emphysema, not the cause.

By acting on the elastic tissue of the lungs, male hormones can prevent chronic emphysema and the shortness of breath associated with aging. The result will be more effective if treatment begins at the appearance of the first symptoms.

23

Metamorphoses of the Silhouette

Abdominal Bloating

The man with an androgenic disease of andropause tends to "inflate," and his silhouette changes (figure 13, page 119).

The abdominal volume, already overloaded with fat, increases further due to the accumulation of large amounts of gas in the digestive tract. Distension is capricious. At first, it appears temporarily. The buttocks inflate first, then, with years, the belly. In men, the abdomen swells first, then, with years, the buttocks. The stomach remains distended.

Gradually, the distension reproduces each day and intensifies during the day. In the evening, swelling peaks, then disappears during the night. Lastly, the belly remains distended permanently, almost simulating pregnancy. A telling characteristic is that this distension does not reabsorb after eliminating gas and stools.

Digested food and the accompanying gases must cross eight meters of the intestine, on average, before being evacuated by the contraction of an important muscle*. In ageing men, intestinal muscles degenerate due to insufficient secretion of male hormones (chapter 13). It follows the atonality of the intestinal muscle fibers, which become unable to contract normally. Consequently, distension becomes permanent.

---

* The motor system of the digestive tract consists of the musculature of the small and large intestines. The small intestine measures approximately 6.5 meters and comprises fifteen to sixteen intestinal loops. It is made of a surface layer with longitudinal muscle fibers and a deep layer with circular fibers.
The length of the large intestine is 1.5 meters, on average. Like the small intestine, it is composed of two muscular layers.

Traditional treatment of gas excess in the belly uses drugs that have the property to fix gases. Coal of vegetable origin is still used for this purpose. Once more, this treats the gas excess, a consequence of the distension, not the *atonic intestinal musculature*, the cause of distension. It is common to see the waist circumference of a swollen woman decrease in a few weeks with mesterolone treatment, while the previously observed weight loss has not yet influenced the roundness.

Mesterolone stimulates the bowel muscles of a man with the androgenic disease of andropause.

Breast Hypertrophy

The man secretes small amounts of female hormone and significant amounts of male hormone. Andropause is a world upside down. Man loses not only the attributes of his sexuality but is also gradually feminized. Modifications in sex hormone balance, with a prevalence of female hormones, cause his feminization. In women, the reverse occurs. She normally secretes female hormones and male hormones before menopause. After the balance is disrupted, male hormones appear to predominate. It explains the appearance of a mustache in a woman with menopause.

Female Hormones in Man

A long time ago, male hormones were the only sex hormones existing in men. The doctor proportioned just blood testosterone to make a diagnosis without considering the possible opposing action of the female hormone, which some denied the existence in men.

However, certain testicle tumors secrete the female hormone, and their blood level can also be high in cases of liver cirrhosis. The secretion of female hormones by the testicle is an accepted concept in endocrinology. Estradiol is also a byproduct of testosterone metabolism. The rise in the blood estradiol level is frequent in a man with an androgenic disease of andropause. Its complex mechanism would require a specific book. The excess of female hormone, generally accompanied by disorders of male hormone secretion, intervenes in a series of complications in men: atrophy of the prostate [1], cardiovascular diseases, and sexual dysfunctions.

In a healthy state, a man's mammary glands are rudimentary; the nipple and the areola surrounding it are undeveloped. The appearance of mammary hypertrophy is men's most visible effect of feminization. It does not happen to all men; however, the phenomenon is not so rare. It is enough to observe the sagging chests of older men on a beach.

Gynecomastia* may develop unilaterally or bilaterally. It is often discrete but can sometimes correspond to the volume of the female breast and can even become sensitive and painful. These symptoms always express a significant imbalance of sex hormones in men.

Mammary hypertrophy must be treated from the outset for better therapeutic results. Symptoms answer, in general, to the regularization of sex hormones. The sensitivity disappears in a few days. The softening of the mammary mass occurs over 2 to 3 weeks, and the reduction in mammary volume takes approximately 2 months.

---

* Gynecomastia is the term for the enlargement of the mammary glands in men.

24

Kidney Failure

The kidneys are filtering stations that purify the blood of metabolic waste products. Urea is the principal waste produced from protein degradation. Degeneration provoked by androgenic menopausal disease induces two mechanisms that involve the progressive destruction of the kidneys. Initially, arteriosclerosis of the renal arteries, followed by hypertension in the renal cavities. These two pathologies lead to renal insufficiency and possibly death by uremia.

The renal arteries participate in the degenerative process, spreading gradually throughout the arterial network (see chapter 12). There is a lack of oxygen in renal tissue, which atrophies, leading to a small, sclerotic kidney. Renal sclerosis, in turn, leads to two phenomena that are highly damaging to the organism: one from excess, the other from the default secretion of renal tissue.

Kidney degeneration leads to the release of renin, an enzyme that increases the production of hypertensive hormones. As a result, it worsens hypertension and arteriosclerosis.

Also, the sick kidney cannot secrete the hormone erythropoietin, which stimulates the formation of red blood cells. This phenomenon causes and worsens anemia in men with an androgenic disease of andropause.

By crossing the renal filter, blood removes excess water and waste products from the body, producing urine that flows through the renal cavities before being propelled by the ureters into the bladder. From there, it is emitted outwardly by the urethra.

The urinary tract is a set of flexible systems. Bladder neck fibrosis is a permanent obstacle to urination. Fibrosis destroys not only the bladder but also the elements above it: the ureters, renal cavities, and kidneys.

The bladder reacts to a bladder neck obstruction by initially hypertrophying its musculature, and it becomes completely flaccid over time.

This pathology triggers another, lesser-known pathology: deformation of the ureteral valve (ureterotrigonal valve), which primarily prevents backward flow of urine toward the kidney. This valve initially tightens, but over time, it dislocates. The curious reader will find an explanation I did fifty years ago, which is easy to assimilate [1].

The deformation of the ureteral valve impedes urine flow toward the bladder. This phenomenon causes hypertension in the renal cavities, with subsequent specific disorders.

Renal colic, generally due to a ureter obstruction by a calculus, is very painful. When there is a prostatic obstruction, the ureteral musculature contracts at its terminal segment in the bladder, causing renal colic in the absence of a calculus* This little-known phenomenon explains certain cases of renal colic whose cause is not evident. It is necessary to consider it in cases of recurrent renal colic and bilateral renal colic (figures 20, 21). The ideal urea level in the blood is from twenty-five to thirty milligrams per hundred milliliters of plasma. When the urinary tract is obstructed, pressure in the renal cavities increases, impairing filtration and purification.

---

* Colic is a pain occurring in the form of violent cramping, felt in the internal organs of the belly.

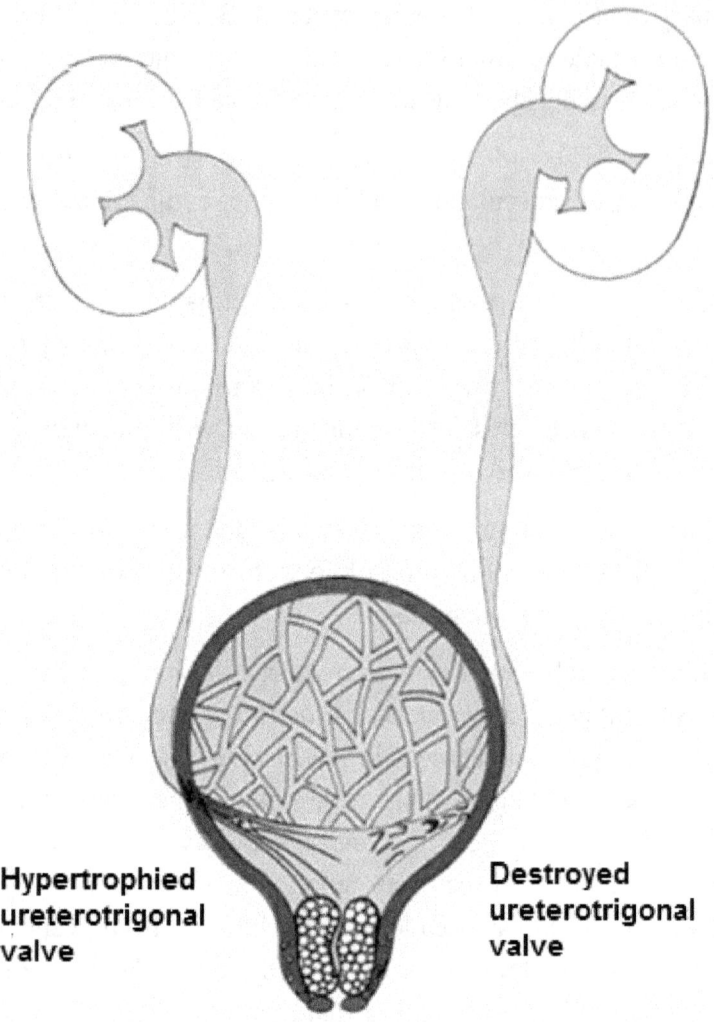

Fig. 20

The prostatic obstruction triggers a reaction in the ureteral musculature. The ureterotrigonal valve is destroyed. Initially, the ureterotrigonal valve hypertrophies, impeding urine flow (on the left). The ureter dilates upstream. The kidney is damaged gradually. The musculature of the ureterotrigonal valve is then displaced. The urine flows back into the dilated ureter (on the right). The kidney is destroyed gradually.

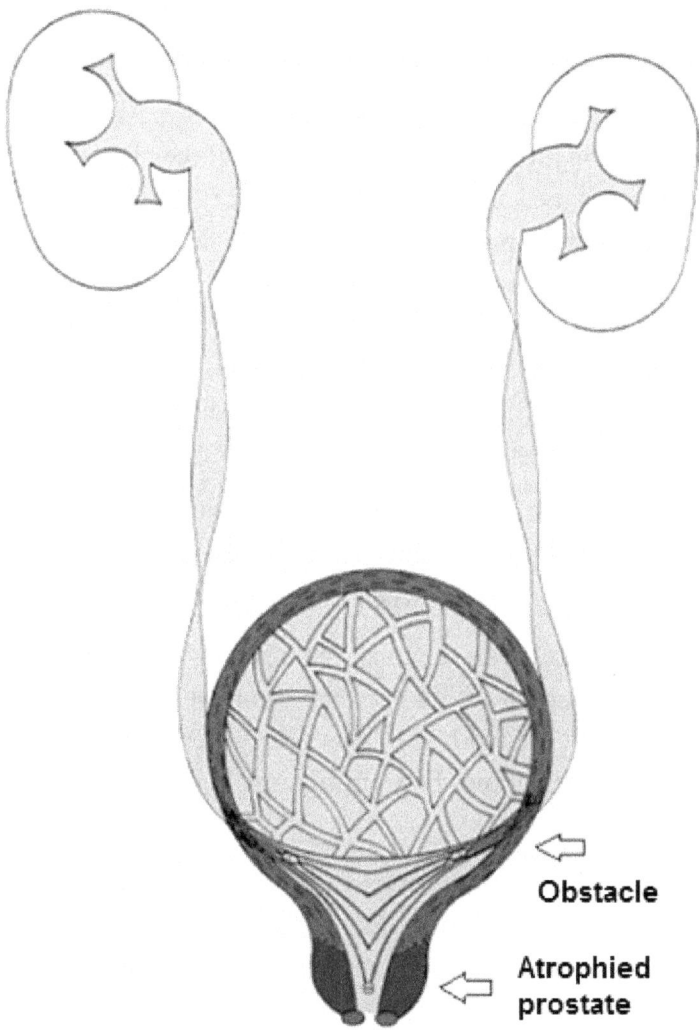

Fig. 21

Atrophy and sclerosis of the bladder neck constitute an obstacle to urination. The vesical muscle reacts and hypertrophies. The ureterotrigonal musculature also thickens. The diameter of the intravesical ureter narrows, and the ureters dilate upstream.

A certain amount of urea circulates in the general circulation, increasing its concentration in the blood, thereby explaining the urea level's progressive rise.

Renal degradation progresses gradually, even if the prostate obstruction is not continuous, because the urinary tract's flexible system distends, compromising the propulsion of urine. In the normal state, the urinary tract must always be free. An obstacle to the flow of urine, apparently undeveloped, constitutes an abnormal resistance that, over time, leads to the destruction of the kidneys. This concept is not always understood. It is, however, essential because obstruction of the urinary tract, even moderate, is incompatible with a long life.

It is necessary to be wary of urea levels that oscillate permanently around forty milligrams per hundred milliliters of plasma. A complete urological checkup is needed when the urea level exceeds this limit.

If the prostate obstruction remains, the urine that cannot be evacuated mixes with blood, and a high concentration causes uremia. The term *uremia* refers to a breakdown of the kidney's excretory function, and the blood urea rises above fifty milligrams per hundred milliliters of plasma.

Death by uremia is relatively peaceful. The patient falls asleep, with urea having a gradual onset like sleeping pills. By making this observation, the idea came to manufacture barbiturates* from urea. The soothing properties of urea explain tiredness and disorders of memory and creativity when its level in the blood starts to rise. These symptoms constitute a real alarm bell.

---

* A barbiturate is an acid whose derivatives are used as sedatives (e.g., Veronal, Gardenal).

Despite a standard health evaluation, migraines and giddiness, with or without accompanying tiredness, must make one think of hypertension in the renal cavities, a generally ignored and unresearched pathology.

Ureters and renal cavities under excessive tension cause turbid reflexes of intestinal contraction. Impaired digestion and distension of the belly are very frequent. One needs this knowledge to avoid taking unnecessary digestive powders over the years. A blocked urinary tract causes water retention. It can reach several liters and cause leg edema. Conserving 2 or 3 liters of water is already significant. It appears in the places where the skin is thinnest. The swelling of the eyelids must draw attention.

A simple blood test can diagnose renal insufficiency. One can then take an X-ray of the urinary tract (intravenous urography) to assess its condition after injecting an iodinated solution into the arm. A few minutes later, it penetrates the urinary tract and shows characteristic anomalies.

Prostate obstacles and sclerosis of the renal arteries cause progressive renal failure in men with an androgenic disease of andropause.

Hearing Loss and Vision Troubles

The sound that strikes the tympanum is transmitted in the ear by a chain of tiny bones articulated between them. Deprived of male hormones, they degenerate like the whole bone tissue. The weakening of hearing announces impending deafness.

Vision Troubles

The most frequent vision pathologies are as follows:

- Presbyopia
- Cataract
- Glaucoma
- Retinal detachment
- Age-related macular degeneration (AMD)

The vision adaptation depends on a whole system of muscles whose tonicity is necessary for correct vision. The generalized involution of the muscles at the time of andropause does not spare ocular tissues. Eye troubles that appear around age forty-five signal hormonal decline.

If one recognizes the importance of male hormones in the arterial network, can one neglect preventive hormonal treatment? Eye troubles in men with an androgenic disease of andropause result from critical vascular modifications, sclerosis phenomena, and glucose and calcium disturbances. They are the consequences of insufficient secretion of male hormones.

Vision loss in older people is generally a manifestation of arteriosclerosis (chapter 14). Tiny eye arteries are sclerosed progressively. Arteriosclerosis is caused by the lack of androgens [1]. In 1998, I advised a seventy-year-old woman who had experienced hemorrhagic losses caused by an "unnecessary hormone replacement therapy" (HRT) to check her male hormones. Unfortunately, she followed her attending physician's advice to do nothing. Later, within years, she developed retinal detachment and is now almost blind.

HRT and Hearing Loss

Hearing problems are common among older people, and centers for hearing studies are increasing as the population ages.

Unnecessary hormone replacement therapy (HRT) in women provokes a decrease in androgen secretion. Consequently, arteriosclerosis and age-related diseases develop. Also, HRT promotes breast cancer [2].

Extensive research demonstrated that women who receive HRT lose more hearing than untreated women. Thus, they must escape monolithic medical practices by using traditional HRT.

The hearing results from the action of a whole series of muscles activating a series of ossicles. The lack of testosterone leads to widespread muscle atrophy, and the ear muscles are no exception. It is the same for the ear's ossicles, altered by a lack of testosterone.

In 2017, Curhan and colleagues from the Channing Division of Network Medicine, Department of Medicine, Brigham and Women's Hospital, Harvard Medical School, Boston, Massachusetts, demonstrated that oral HRT was associated with a higher risk of hearing loss among postmenopausal women. In addition, a longer duration of use was associated with a higher risk [3].

26

Immune Deficiency, AIDS, and Cancer

The media frequently announces accidents causing hip fractures in a famous older man, specifying that it will take them many months of readjustment after hip replacement surgery. Then, one or two years later, the media announces the death of the same famous older man following a lung infection. The chronology from hip fracture to the end, caused by a lung infection, is common.

Testosterone stimulates immunity. The reduction in androgens decreases lymphocyte production, thereby promoting the development of infection and cancer [1–3]. Testosterone is an immune modulator, a property that allows the body to resist some disease-causing agents.

AIDS

Androgens can be more critical in patients with AIDS, especially when they are weak, experience pain with physical effort, and have low lymphocyte levels. This protective action of androgens on the globules was shown in 1997 by S. A. Klein and his collaborators. A thirty-seven-year-old man was in an extreme state of leanness. After three weeks' treatment with an androgen (1 alpha-dihydrotestosterone), the destruction of lymphocytes was reduced by 34 percent compared to the beginning of the therapy. At the same time, his general and nutritional condition was remarkably improved [4].

In 2009, a publication from the Program on Developmental Endocrinology and Genetics of the National Institutes of Health in Bethesda, Maryland, reported the prolongation of lymphocyte telomeres under the influence of androgens [5]. Telomeres protect chromosomes from damage, and a shorter leukocyte telomere length is a marker of advancing biological age. Telomerase is involved in telomere length. New studies about hormonal links with telomerase and stem cells are now necessary for older men.

COVID-19 and Viral Infections

Immunodeficiency is more common after the age of 60. The recent COVID-19 pandemic has demonstrated this. The average age of death due to infection was around 80 years.

Life expectancy in the most developed countries in terms of public health is 82 years. Unfortunately, many deaths are caused by infections promoted by deficient immunity at this age.

The decline in immunity after age 40 depends on decreases in testosterone secretion [1-2-3-4-5] and melatonin secretion after age 50. Recent studies have demonstrated the value of melatonin in treating severe COVID-19 cases, with excellent results [6-7]. In conclusion, to prevent infections associated with ageing immunity, it is desirable to address hormonal deficiencies after 40. Daily testosterone and melatonin production can be measured. Hormone compensation is inexpensive.

Cancer

According to the World Health Organization, cancer is a significant cause of death globally, causing 9,555,027 deaths in 2018.

One area of immunity research concerns the prevention and treatment of tumors. Today, considerable progress has been made in comprehending cancer's mechanisms, thanks to James Allison and Tasuku Honjo. They received the Nobel Prize in Physiology or Medicine in 2018 for their discovery of a cancer treatment that inhibits negative immune regulation. Immunotherapy is regarded more and more as an alternative therapy. Specific tumors can even be cured with treatments that harness the tools of immunity. The pharmaceutical industry has already brought to market anticancer drugs approved by the US Food and Drug Administration (FDA).

Preventing tumors can benefit from melatonin treatment, according to the work of Russel J. Reiter of the University of Texas Health Science Center at San Antonio [8].

Without prevention, the future of older people is either degeneration due to arteriosclerosis and Alzheimer's disease or the development of tumors. We have already seen that arteriosclerosis can be prevented. Its preventive treatment with mesterolone as early as forty is decisive. This result will be even more impressive if melatonin is taken simultaneously with mesterolone, as it prevents tumor development [9].

27

Depression

A man with the androgenic disease of andropause sees a complete upheaval of his mental structures because the brain, a large consumer of male hormones, is not stimulated and degenerates. Depression settles in and causes the appearance of many negative symptoms that will affect daily life. The World Health Organization estimates that experiences of depression affect more than 350,000,000 individuals each year [1]. Fifty percent of doctor visits are due to this disease, whose cause is curiously unknown. The action of male hormones on the nervous system should make one reflect that.

Today, we see the importance of male hormones for nerve cells and behavior. A whole work would be necessary to develop the subject; studies are numerous and exceed the framework of this book. But the following sections will reveal an unexpected aspect of sex hormones, which control not only our sexuality but also our thoughts, our moods, and our behaviors.

Studies have shown that sex hormones are highly concentrated in the nervous system. The demonstration was made in rats by injecting dihydrotestosterone labeled with radioactive isotopes. Histological cuts showed localization of the labeled molecules in various nervous structures of sacrificed animals. Brain cells, the cerebellum, the spinal cord, and cranial nerve cells contain potent male hormone molecules. Male hormones are primarily concentrated in the motor cells that control movement. Female hormones are mainly present in sensitive nerve cells.

Male hormones are also present in the other brain components, such as the arteries and ventricles*

The presence of male hormones in the brain is vital, as one can question their role in degenerative nervous system diseases when they are insufficient.

There are also cerebral centers of sexuality. Their sensitivity to the action of male and female sex hormones explains the differences in sexual behaviors. Behavior depends, consequently, on the effect of sex hormones on the nerve cells.

Aggressiveness, Predominance, Libido

All parents know the difficult puberty period among boys when high quantities of male hormones permeate all structures of their bodies. Disturbed opposition and aggressiveness of teenagers are psychological signs of natural biological evolution. Unfortunately for the parents and the teenagers, it is inevitable and constitutes one rather painful period of three or four years of incomprehension and confrontations.

The aggressive impulses caused by male hormones were the subject of several scientific studies that show the concordance between male hormone levels and aggression.

Harold Persky and his collaborators studied the reactions of men subjected to specific constraining personality tests, making it possible to quantify the various degrees of anxiety, depression, and aggressiveness [2]. They studied men into two age groups. The first group comprises young men with an average age of around 22 years. The second group includes men having an average age of forty-five.

---

* The ventricles are cerebral cavities that contain cerebrospinal fluid.

The plasmatic testosterone levels and the daily testosterone production are given to everyone before and during the personality tests.

Correlation of plasmatic testosterone level of two groups of men subjected to aggressiveness tests	
	Testosterone level in Nanograms/100 mL
Young men	685
Older men	404

Table 10

According to Persky and colleagues [2].

The comparison between the two groups is particularly impressive. Young men show reactions of hostility proportional to their testosterone levels, the most aggressive having the highest levels. One can even predict the reaction's intensity based on hormonal levels. Reactions in older men are independent of their male hormone levels, probably because of insufficient secretion.

One showed the relationship between male hormone levels and the aggressiveness of hockey players [3]. Factors such as a leader's temperament, competitiveness, offensive play, tolerance of frustration, use of force at the time of body contact, responses to threats, and total aggressiveness were quantified on a scale from 1 to 5.

The authors noted a positive correlation between the importance of aggressive reactions and plasmatic testosterone levels. The violent answer to a threat corresponds to the highest quantities of male hormones.

Statistics of mortality caused by accidents in the United States are also edifying if one compares the mortality rate of women with that of men according to their age [4]. The reading of Table 9 is entirely significant. Men die three times more from violent deaths than women. After sixty-five, having lost their sex hormones and aggressiveness, they support external pressures.

The number of deaths by accidents recorded in the United States in 1982 [4].			
Less than sixty-five years		More than sixty-five years	
Men	Women	Men	Women
54,000	17,000	12,000	11,000

Table 11

In 1975, Robert Rose and his collaborators observed the behaviors of four male monkeys in the presence of thirteen females. The group's relations cause significant variations: testosterone levels rise gradually in the dominant male and fall by 80% in the other three. Suppose the dominant male is introduced into another group of monkeys led by a leader he cannot dominate. In that case, his testosterone level is reduced during the first week of confrontation to reach 80 percent of its initial values six weeks later [5]. This phenomenon prevents mortal combat and allows males to coexist within the same social organization. If he remains subject to the dominating male presence, the dominated monkey secretes fewer male hormones and remains flexible and apprehensive, with a weak libido. It is enough to separate him from the leader to recover, at the same time, a normal testicular secretion, sex drive, and aggressiveness.

The predominance of men also depends on testicular secretion. Therefore, the testosterone level was given to thirty-six prisoners divided into three groups of twelve men according to their degree of predominance and subjected to personality tests for aggressiveness [6].

The first group comprises men who have shown chronic aggressiveness: violent physical aggression, worsened attacks, crimes, and still uttering aggressive words and threats despite imprisonment.

The second group comprises socially dominant men occupying a raised situation in the social hierarchy, white-collar criminals imprisoned for robbery, drug racket, or illicit money.

Lastly, the third group comprises nonviolent prisoners who are socially non-dominant.

Correlation of the plasmatic testosterone level and the degree of predominance in man	
Degree of predominance	Testosterone level in nanograms/100 mL
Unaggressive men	599
Socially aggressive men	836
Aggressive men	1010

Table 12

According to Ehrenkrantz J., Bliss, E., and Sheard, M. H. [6].

The experiment shows that the most aggressive have the highest testosterone levels and the least aggressive have the lowest levels

(Table 10). The socially dominant men have an average level of dominance. Hormonal levels are characteristic of each individual and vary little over the course of a day. The most aggressive men are remarkably insensitive to anxiety [6].

In tennis players who have played a match for "honor," the testosterone levels are lower in losers. On the other hand, testosterone levels rise in students receiving their diplomas during a public ceremony [7]. The rise in social status, meaning more considerable merit and getting a feeling of joy and deep completion, is translated in man by increasing the secretion of his male hormones.

Male hormone secretion conditions the intensity of the libido. When they are secreted in excess, they cause hypersexuality. The phenomenon is sometimes so intense that it causes sexual crimes. Formerly, criminals were castrated. Fortunately, today, there are drugs able to neutralize the actions of male hormones.

Lederer [8] described an exemplary case of hypersexuality: "M. C., a professor at a university, got married when he was twenty-two years old, for opportunity reasons, to a person he loved. While having regular sexual intercourse with his wife, to whom he gave five children, he quickly took a mistress, with whom he had almost daily relationships. That was not enough for him. He still had relationships with other women (up to two or three times per day). If necessary, he contacted a young man, leading to several serious problems with the judicial authorities. At the time of one of those, he was addressed to me. He had the external attitude of a hypersexual individual: the glance shining, a marked chin, an extraordinarily strong pilosity of the face and the body, and extremely developed genitals. While managing this man with a drug neutralizing testosterone (cyproterone acetate), things returned to normal."

Neutralizing male hormones produces psychological relaxation, and aggression gives way to serenity. However, the anti-male hormone treatment managed with substantial amounts causes impotence and sexual failure.

Lack of Creativity, Memory Loss, Reduced Dynamism, and Behavioral Problems

The mentally healthy man can adapt to the various significantly changing situations in the external world. His relationship to the entourage, the ambient conditions, and the world he lives in imply various relational aspects related to thoughts, mood, intuitive life, aspirations and will, behavior, and self-awareness. These faculties depend mainly on brain impregnation by sex hormones. Therefore, the man with an androgenic disease of andropause gradually loses his mental faculties in a depressive context. Mauvais-Jarvis and de Lignières estimate that the endocrinology of depression should be one of the most urgent research topics; the incidence of the lack of male hormones in a man's depressive disease seems exceptionally high [9].

Depression and lack of male hormones in men		
Men consulting for impotence	Number of cases	Plasmatic testosterone in nanograms/100 mL
Depressed	8	205
Non-depressed	9	645

Table 13

According to Lignières and Mauvais-Jarvis [9].

All mental faculties diminish gradually when male hormones are lacking. For example, creativity decreases in artists, painters, sculptors, writers, and so forth, and then disappears. Hormonal treatment restarts their creative faculties, making their works more durable and beautiful.

In an ordinary man, the capacity to fix memory varies with age. A three-year-old child remembers a series of three numbers. At four years, the child retains four. Between six and eight years, the child memorizes five numbers; at ten years, six; and at fourteen years, a series of seven. The number of series that a healthy adult can remember hovers around 7 digits.

Traditional treatment of depression uses antidepressant drugs. Monoamine oxidase inhibitors, a class of cerebral enzymes, are commonly prescribed. However, they are not always well supported because they can cause giddiness, headaches, nausea, and constipation. Interestingly, *testosterone is a natural inhibitor of monoamine oxidase*. Therefore, the disappearance of depressive symptoms can be achieved within a few days, once the brain contains male hormones [10].

Memory loss is one of the primary symptoms of andropause. Curiously, recent events are initially forgotten, whereas past images remain in memory. The man forgets the answer he received to the questions he repeats, sometimes on several occasions, without realizing it. Under these conditions, giving courses or making review articles becomes challenging. The man with androgen deficiency (andropause) cannot fix his ideas. The progressive loss of his mental faculties can make him unemployed and unable to reintegrate into society.

Memory loss is one of the primary symptoms of the androgenic disease of andropause. Curiously, recent facts are forgotten, whereas past images remain in memory. Under these conditions, continuing in one's occupation can become complicated. Men with the androgenic disease of andropause are unable to retain their ideas. A progressive loss of mental faculties can result in these men becoming unemployed and unable to reintegrate into society.

In the morning, the man with an androgen deficiency (andropause) rises tired. During the day, he drags. At the limit, he is tired of being tired, with all his cerebral structures lacking male hormones. He becomes unable to use the whole of his intellectual faculties and does not perceive any goal to realize. "To act" and "to want" are lost concepts because vital energy has disappeared. Instinctively, he knows that the countdown has started and that there is nothing to hope for anymore. How often I've heard, "I am tired," "I quit the business," "My job is rotten, I do not know what to do," or "I thought about running for election, but I gave up." I've heard the same men say, after hormonal treatment, "To give up my business? I do not think of it anymore. On the contrary, I created a new one," or, "I reconsidered my job; I am leaving for new horizons," or, "Finally, I ran and won the election." Those results are something completely refreshing.

There is no sexual instinct without male hormones. The absence of libido can occur suddenly; generally, it settles down gradually, and certain men accept it as they get used to it. Others seek to be reassured. They think that the phenomenon is momentary. Then they begin looking for all kinds of excuses. Little by little, concern appears. Sexual intercourse becomes increasingly rare; months pass without any sexual desire. The repercussions in the couple's relationship are inevitable, especially when the partner is younger. Comprehension quickly leads to suspicions: "He misleads me," or, worse, "He does not like me anymore."

Consequently, the vicious circle of mutual incomprehension starts with, on the one hand, an increasingly ice-cold woman and, on the other side, a woman haunted by a fear of failure due to lack of desire. With time, the situation becomes intolerable, even dramatic, and inevitably leads to the lovers' separation. Of course, all of that would have fallen into place if the lack of hormones had not worsened the situation.

A man must unceasingly protect himself from external aggressions by mobilizing his hormonal balance controlled by the brain. The mechanism is always the same in all the circumstances of life: loss of a loved one, unemployment, bankruptcy, surgical procedure, burns, and conflict without exit. All body reactions to aggression were brilliantly described and proven by the Canadian physiologist Hans Selye under the *general adaptation syndrome*, which is generally called the *effects of stress*.

Everything starts with an alarm reaction that mobilizes the hormones of the suprarenal glands (cortisol and adrenaline), which are the hormones of urgency. At the same time, the secretion of male hormones rises, increasing aggressiveness and providing the energy reserves necessary for combat or escape (by increasing the muscles' metabolism). Then, if stress is prolonged or reproduced at too high a frequency, the secretion of male hormones falls, leading to depression, with the incapacity to react. Under these conditions, a man with an androgenic disease of andropause constitutes prey to stress because he cannot mobilize his male hormones in enough quantity.

Morbid unhappiness without apparent cause is a natural consequence of the androgenic disease of andropause. Nevertheless, there is a gross disproportion between the futility of the reason and the intensity of sadness and gloomy mood. Discouragement, dislike, and pessimism are parts of daily life, which seem dull, gray, and stripped of direction.

Concern leads to anxiety, possibly with fear of the surrounding world.

Melancholy of men with an androgenic disease of andropause is always present if not accompanied by various disorders. Men complaining about sexual conditions due to age very often take antidepressant drugs, their sexual failures being attributed, wrongly, to mood disorders. It is not so much the depression that should be erased, but the pressure put on the organism, which is different. Male hormones have the particularity of stimulating cerebral and sexual functions simultaneously.

Depression also appears with disorders of self-awareness. The feeling of not being oneself, of losing standing, or of no longer belonging to humanity inevitably leads to withdrawal, isolation, and the sense of living under a bell. Inability to communicate causes ruptures with the external world, which appears increasingly hostile. The situation becomes complicated because of people's incomprehension at home or at work, especially when nothing explains the odd, silent behavior. Charges are concise: "And yet he has everything to be happy about"; "He is a shirker"; "He has something in mind." Consequently, depression worsens; black thoughts appear and sometimes lead to suicide. Unfairly accusing the weak always seemed unbearable to me, mainly because the accusations often come from beings who are only strong in front of weak ones.

Bob, 56, just lost his job. He was unemployed and had no hope of finding a job. He was depressed and unable to react. To his misfortune, his virility disappeared. Despairing, he consulted his doctor. At first glance, this doctor saw an overweight man with a prominent belly under a gray waistcoat. His thick neck appeared too short. His face was bloated. His falling eyelids gave him an air of false somnolence. The diagnosis was already made: androgenic disease of andropause. Bob confirmed back pain, difficulty with digestion, depressive mood, and impotence. A simple blood control confirmed the diagnosis: the rise in cholesterol, diabetes, and, inevitably, low male hormones. It would be necessary to lose ten kilos and to take male hormones. Bob was skeptical; he believed that his depression was the cause of his misfortune, but, after all, the treatment seemed relatively simple to him, so he would do what was necessary. Three months later, he went back to his doctor. Bob lost five kilos. The blood examinations improved; he found his manhood again, decided to create a new job, and realized that his disgrace and depression resulted from the biochemical deterioration caused by his insufficiency of male hormones. He subsequently understood that he would carefully monitor his food intake and hormone levels. Bob was again young. It was only the beginning.

In 2012, the Department of Urology at Baylor College of Medicine, Houston, Texas, published a study in which substitution therapy with testosterone can reduce the symptoms of depression in men with low levels of male hormones, like in middle-aged men taking antidepressants [11].

In 2012, the Chinese Medical Newspaper published a work by researchers at the Department of Urology at Beijing University People's Hospital in China. They showed that testosterone improves Chinese men's psychological distress and quality of health. In addition, those patients presented late hypogonadism [12].

Late hypogonadism is defined classically as insufficiency of testosterone secretion when the testosterone level is between two hundred fifty and three hundred nanograms per one hundred milliliters of blood. This observation is not rare in men beyond seventy. It is the *final stage of the* androgenic disease andropause, which generally begins at 40 and sometimes even earlier. This ageing disease results from reduced secretion of male hormones (testosterone and dihydrotestosterone). The diagnosis is founded on the study of the complete metabolism of androgens. During the first years of the disease (for example, between forty and sixty-five years), the blood testosterone level can be higher than 300 nanograms per 100 milliliters of plasma. In contrast, studies of daily androgen secretion show insufficient production. This study determines the levels of hormonal precursors, the proportions of androgen hormones, and their metabolites in urine over 24 hours.

In the 1990s, doctors thought dehydroepiandrosterone (DHEA) intake could overcome depression. DHEA is a testosterone precursor available freely in drugstores in the United States.

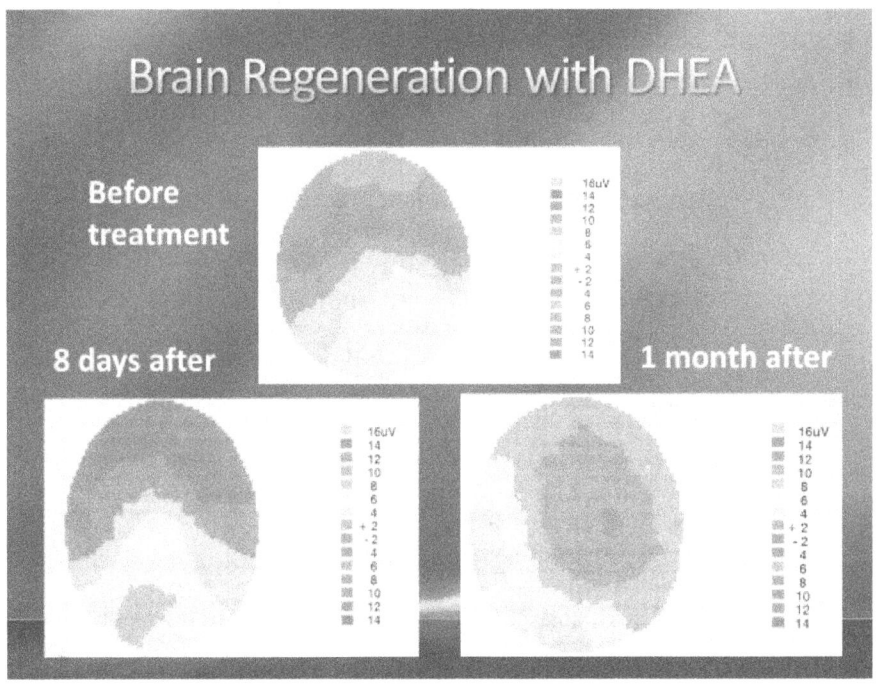

Fig. 22

Based on Bonnet and Brown [13].

In 1990, a study was undertaken by the Department of Psychiatry of New York University School of Medicine in which a depressed woman was given considerable DHEA. The patient received 12.5 mg/kg/day (low dose) or 37 mg/kg/day (high dose) for two years. The patient weighed seventy kilos. With these incredibly high doses, DHEA converts into high testosterone levels in the blood, resulting in a rapid improvement in brain activity. Before treatment, the brain scan recordings, eight days after and one month later, showed significant improvement (figure 22). Such doses of DHEA are inappropriate and dangerous in women and men. But it is remarkable to note the rapid improvement of brain activity.

Their brain scans will also show this improvement with physiological doses of safe mesterolone in depressed men. This study remains to be done and will be of the highest interest.

The problems with the use of DHEA are as follows:

- It is a chemical substance that is a precursor of hormones.
- The administered doses transform it into various substances (e.g., testosterone and estradiol, a female hormone) [14].
- It is not converted directly into dihydrotestosterone (the potent sex hormone for men and women).
- According to the administered doses, it slows down the pituitary gland by producing contradictory hormonal substances.
- It does not correspond to a well-defined pathology.
- It transforms testosterone into estradiol, a female hormone that is a proliferative hormone.
- It should not be sold without a medical prescription.
- It is not the treatment for the androgenic disease of andropause.

In 2018, Positron Emission Tomography (PET) was a non-invasive imaging tool used to evaluate the effects of hormonal therapy on specific downstream processes in the brain. [15].

The production of male hormones decreases gradually and continuously over the years in men and women, causing a weakened and depressed older adult. However, this production shortfall can occur within a few months.

28

Parkinson's Disease

A biochemical substance partly orders our movements. It is dopamine secreted by specialized cells located in the center of the base of the brain (the *substantia nigra, or locus niger*). These cells no longer secrete dopamine; the musculature solidifies and is prone to shaking when destroyed.

The Frozen Drug Addicts

William Langston, a neurologist at Santa Clara Valley Medical Center in Northern California, was stunned by the arrival at his office of a motionless young man, as if frozen mute, with large open eyes that did not blink.

One can understand the stupefaction of the other doctors consulted, who had never seen such a case before. By examining the young man's girlfriend, Langston, and his fellow neurologist, Phil Ballard, he noted that she was in the same frozen state as the young man. They suspected a connection between the two cases.

By chance, Ballard attended a meeting arranged by his neurologist friend, James Tetrud, who told him he had seen two similar cases during his consultation.

The four "frozen" people were heroin addicts. Langston went on television to alert the community to the existence of illegally tainted heroin sold on the street. Following this, a spectator announced two other cases. Six individuals were "frozen."

Langston got samples of the remaining substance that the victims had injected. Analyses of the drug sold as heroin showed that it was a toxic synthetic product, MPTP* which causes permanent symptoms of Parkinson's disease by destroying specific neurons in the black substance of the brain. Studies using this molecule are undertaken in monkeys.

The story of the frozen drug addicts was told with passion by William Langston and Jon Palfreman, a medical writer, in the book *The Case of the Frozen Addicts: How the Solution of an Extraordinary Medical Mystery Has Spawned a Revolution in the Understanding and Treatment of Parkinson's Disease* [1]. When a frozen addict dies, the autopsy shows the destruction of the cells secreting dopamine in the brain.

When the cells that secrete dopamine die or are damaged, one sees the appearance of motor disorders of progressive evolution. Parkinson's disease usually begins at age forty-five or fifty (ages for the beginning of the menopausal illness) or later. It is the second-most-frequent neurodegenerative disease after Alzheimer's disease.

Parkinson's disease provokes motor symptoms (e.g., shaking, muscular rigidity, slow movements) and nonmotor symptoms (e.g., constipation, disturbed sleep, urination emergencies, frigidity, dizzy spells, tiredness, depression, memory disorders). This disease results from a deficiency in dopamine production by specialized cells deep in the brain. One cause of the destruction of cells that produce dopamine is that they no longer receive blood due to arteriosclerosis [2] (chapter 14). Testosterone could play a determining role in biochemistry, even in the cells producing dopamine [3], or by improving blood circulation to these cells. An exciting area of research is the daily androgen production in women with Parkinson's disease. Also, treatment with

---

* MPTP: 1-methyl, 4-phenyl, 1, 2, 3, 6-tetrahydro pyridine.

androgens will decrease the tendency toward depression and limit the need to take "antidepressants."

Normal Production of Androgens	Insufficient Production of Androgens
↓	↓
Tiny, permeable arteries	Tiny, blocked arteries
↓	↓
Normal cells secreting dopamine	Cells secreting dopamine destroyed
↓	↓
Normal production of dopamine	Insufficient production of dopamine
↓	↓
Normal movements	Shaking

Parkinson's and Alzheimer's disease are also observed in patients undergoing surgery or radiation therapy for prostate cancer. Doctors have suppressed testosterone in one way or another, as was done fifty years ago. This suppression no longer corresponds to current scientific data [4-5]. However, the best androgen supplementation is mesterolone. Unlike testosterone, this hormone does not turn into estradiol, a proliferative hormone. In addition, this treatment depends on each patient's singularity. [6].

Given the full extent of the disasters caused by arterial rigidity, can one neglect their prevention with androgen hormones?

Dementias and Alzheimer's Disease

Alzheimer's Disease in Short

Dementias result from a progressive reduction in blood flow to the brain, leading to atrophy and destruction of brain tissue. In addition, those phenomena provoke secondary lesions (senile plaques), amyloid deposits, and immune reactions in Alzheimer's disease, a neurodegenerative pathology.

Alzheimer's disease is generally the result of poor blood flow to certain brain regions where memory is concentrated: the amygdala and the hippocampus.

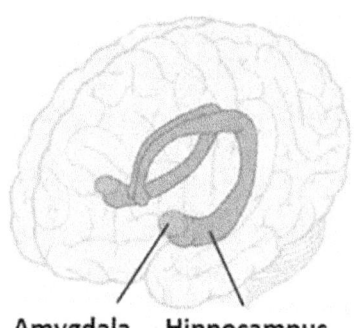

Fig. 23

Amygdala and hippocampus in the depths of the brain.

Arteriosclerosis is a disease of ageing that causes a progressive narrowing of the brain arteries. This phenomenon starts around age forty and will affect everyone over time. Thus, the prevention of the pathology known as Alzheimer's disease must start around age forty.

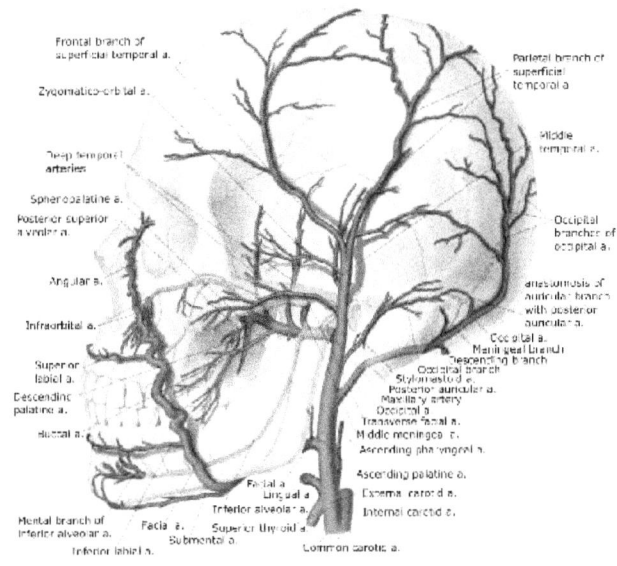

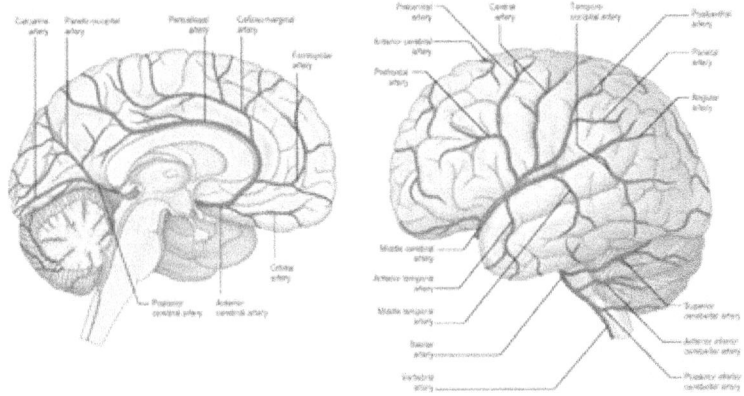

Fig. 24

Normal brain arteries.

When an arterial branch becomes clogged, the tissue of the irrigated area is destroyed.

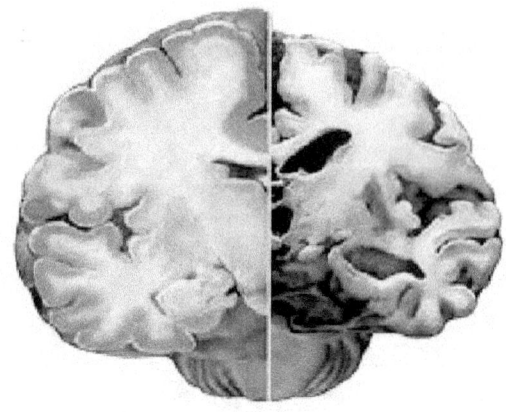

Fig. 25

Left: Healthy brain. Right: Alzheimer's brain tissue—the final stage.

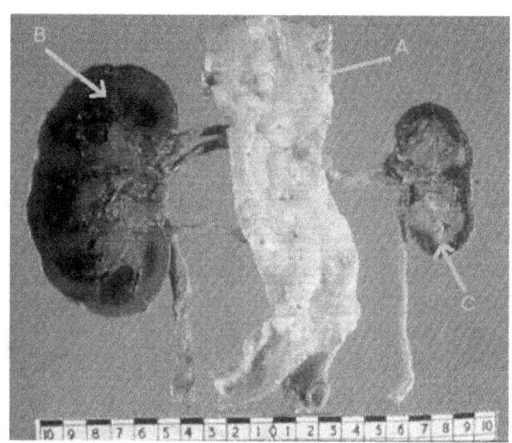

Fig. 26

Left (B): Healthy kidney. Right (C): Atrophied kidney following arterial stenosis and thus a progressive diminution of blood flow in the organ, producing atrophy and destroying the kidney tissue.

Treatment of secondary lesions (senile plaques), amyloid deposits, and immune reactions is hazardous and abandoned [1].

Arteriosclerosis is a disease of ageing that causes narrowing of the arteries. This phenomenon starts around age forty and may be responsible for vascular disorders of various organs (hypertension, Parkinson's disease, vision and hearing troubles, etc.)

The progressive diminution of blood flow to the brain leads to atrophy and destruction of brain tissue.

Arteriosclerosis is a disease of ageing that produces a progressive hardening and narrowing of the brain arteries. Over time, arteriosclerosis destroys the entire brain. The brain with Alzheimer's (figure 25) is final.

As noted, the destruction of the brain starts around age forty and will reach everybody with time; thus, the prevention of dementia must start around age forty.

Arteriosclerosis, whose cause is classically unknown, develops randomly in different areas of the brain. Arteriosclerosis of the cerebral arteries is a general phenomenon associated with dementia.

Depending on the location of the vascular involvement generally associated with dementia, the symptoms will be those of Alzheimer's, vascular dementia, or Parkinson's disease.

Different areas of the brain can be affected. At first, destruction affects specific regions. For example, Alzheimer's disease is a type of dementia characterized by progressive memory loss associated with secondary lesions (senile plaques), amyloid deposits, and immune reactions. This pathology affects the amygdala and hippocampus, located deep in the brain.

For example, tremors are characteristic of Parkinson's disease. This pathology affects the substantia nigra, a midbrain basal ganglia structure.

Over time, arteriosclerosis destroys the entire brain.

How to Stop It?

Again, the destruction of the brain starts around age forty and will reach everybody with time; thus, the prevention of dementia must start around age forty.

A drug can only reach the diseased areas of the brain if the cerebral arteries are permeable. Research should start there.

Therefore, for natural molecules such as hormones or drug molecules to reach brain cells, it is essential first to keep the cerebral arteries healthy, which is the proper treatment for preventing diseases of ageing [2].

Alzheimer's Disease Facts and Figures

Twenty years or more before symptoms appear, the brain changes of Alzheimer's may begin.

In the United States, 5.8 million Americans live with Alzheimer's dementia.

Deaths from Alzheimer's increased by 145 percent between 2000 and 2017.

The estimated cost of Alzheimer's and other dementias, including costs of health care, long-term care, and hospice, totaled $290 billion in 2019 [3].

Dementia Rates

The World Health Organization noted in 2019 that dementia affects about 50 million people worldwide, approximately 60 percent of whom live in low- and middle-income countries. There are about ten million new cases each year. Between 5 and 8 percent of the general population aged sixty or over has dementia at any given time.

The total number of people with dementia will reach 82 million in 2030 and 152 million in 2050. In low- and middle-income countries, the number of people with dementia will continue to increase.

What Is Known

Contrary to popular opinion, brain degeneration does not result in a continuous loss of nerve cells. Instead, the brain loses approximately 10,000 cells per day from the ten billion neurons*. Consequently, the cellular loss represents only 3 percent of nervous cells over eighty years and does not seem responsible for the degeneration. The remaining cells are sufficient. Instead, degeneration results from the atrophy and disappearance of the ramifications that link the nervous cells, enabling them to communicate.

Male Hormones Regenerate Nerve Cells

In the 1970s and 1980s, researchers highlighted the brain's plasticity.

Philippe van den Bosch de Aguilar, a neurobiologist at the Catholic University of Leuven in Belgium, studied the brains of seven generations of rats over 15 years, observing and counting neurons. He noted that the brain's nerve cells develop new nervous terminations at around twenty-four months, a lifetime corresponding to eighty years in man. This study established a new concept: the older brain retains the capacity for reactivity and plasticity.

Dick Swaab from the Netherlands' Institute for Brain Research demonstrated the beneficial effects of testosterone on rats' brains. The microscope indicated that the young rat's nerve cells were well ramified. These ramifications disappeared in the old rat but reappeared

---

* Neuron: a nervous cell generally made up of a body of variable form and equipped with various prolongations, one of which, threadlike and longer than the others, is called the axon.

under testosterone, managed in the form of implants. The phenomenon is most probably the same in humans.

Nervous fibers are surrounded by a myelin* sheath that insulates them and protects them to support the propagation of nerve impulses, like plastic does around electric wires.

Today, it is possible to repair nerve fibers damaged by myelin loss in degenerative brain diseases. In 2013, a group of researchers from different INSERM (the French National Institute of Health and Medical Research) units and various US universities described androgen receptors in the nerve cells of a mouse. These receptors constitute a therapeutic target for myelin repair in nerve cells, which lose this component of their structure when spontaneous myelin repair is no longer possible. This effect is probably due to testosterone's immune, anti-inflammatory, and neuroprotective action [4]. Consequently, it seems logical to me to analyze the androgen production in a woman and a man with nervous system degeneration to manage androgen treatment with total safety. Detection and hormonal treatment are necessary from the onset of primary symptoms to prevent irreversible nerve damage.

Dementias

The World Health Organization (WHO) published the 2012 report "Dementia: A Public Health Priority," which mentions information about dementia [5]. Dementia is a syndrome characterized by deterioration of memory, intellect, behavior, and the capacity to carry out daily activities. Worldwide, there are some 35.6 million people who have dementia. Each year, there are 7.7 million new cases. According to this WHO report, the number of people affected by dementia will triple in 2050, increasing the number of affected individuals to 115 million. Dementia is one of the leading causes of dependence in older

---

* Myelin: a substance made up of fats and proteins.

adults worldwide. Dementia has a physical, psychological, social, and economic impact on nursing staff, families, and society. Six percent of older people over age sixty-five are affected by a variable degree of dementia caused by the deterioration of the nervous ramifications and the appearance of degenerative plaques in the cerebral structures.

Variety of Dementias

There are four subtypes of dementia: Alzheimer's disease, vascular dementia, dementia with Lewy bodies, and frontotemporal dementia. The diagnosis must be interpreted cautiously because clear cases are rarer than mixed pathologies.

Alzheimer's Disease

Alzheimer's disease is the most common cause of dementia. It represents between 60 and 70 percent of the cases of dementia.

Generally Accepted Ideas

Despite a more thorough knowledge of Alzheimer's disease, many generally accepted ideas still circulate on this neurodegenerative pathology, among which are that Alzheimer's disease is a natural consequence of old age or that Alzheimer's disease is a quite specific and incurable degenerative disease. These beliefs do not correspond to reality.

Various Forms of Alzheimer's Disease

The most common form is the nonhereditary or sporadic form. It accounts for 99 percent of cases. The other, very rare, form is the family or hereditary form.

Various Stages of Alzheimer's Disease

Alzheimer's disease passes through multiple phases, which will lead to death in eight to twelve years. The four stages are the initial period, the moderate stage, the severe stage, and the final stage.

Pathological Modifications in the Brain

Alzheimer's disease is characterized by the deposition of senile plaques containing β-amyloid protein and abnormal tangles of nerve fibers in affected cerebral areas.

These anomalies trigger immune responses that exacerbate cellular destruction [6–8].

Recent and Determining Scientific Discoveries

In 1999, researchers at Rockefeller University in New York and Cornell University in New York made an important discovery. Using cultures of nerve cells, they showed that testosterone reduces the secretion of the protein β-amyloid peptide [9].

This study concluded that androgens could protect against the development of Alzheimer's disease.

In 2001, a research team at the University of Western Australia in Perth published the first clinical description of elevated β-amyloid levels in the blood [10]. They showed that chemical castration in men caused a drop in plasma estradiol and testosterone levels parallel to the rise in β-amyloid protein. The *Journal of the American Medical Association* published this capital discovery: "Chemical Andropause and Amyloid-Beta Peptide" (2001, 285: 2195–2196). This study shows that testosterone replacement can prevent or delay Alzheimer's disease.

In 2004, researchers at the University of Southern California studied the brain testosterone content in deceased men in two groups. The first group did not present neuropathology (group controls). The second group suffered from Alzheimer's disease or moderate neuropathology.

This study concluded that the cerebral tissue of patients who had Alzheimer's disease contained significantly less testosterone than the brains of men without a neurophysiological anomaly [11].

In 2008, Emily R. Rosario and Christian J. Pike reviewed scientific publications on Alzheimer's disease [12]. The conclusion of this review was as follows:

Alzheimer's disease shows an abnormal accumulation of the protein β-amyloid in the brain. Recent studies suggest the regulating action of androgens on the β-amyloid protein and the development of Alzheimer's disease. Therapy with androgens may prevent and treat Alzheimer's disease.

In 2011, Emily Rosario and collaborators demonstrated decreased brain levels of androgen and estrogen hormones in men and women during healthy ageing, which may be relevant to the development of Alzheimer's disease [13]. In the same year, an article in the *American Family Physician* noted the small effect of treatment with testosterone on Alzheimer's disease [14]. This conclusion is exact. Indeed, with destroyed nervous tissue, no effective drug exists. However, male hormones effectively prevent Alzheimer's disease before destroying nerve cells.

How to Direct the Treatment of Alzheimer's Disease with Androgens?

The clinical studies carried out to date are remarkable. They highlight the significant impact of testosterone on Alzheimer's disease [9–13]. There are, however, recent publications from eminent researchers who question the effectiveness of androgens in treating Alzheimer's disease [14]. The destruction of nerve cells is always definitive. How to solve these apparent contradictions?

The role of testosterone and androgens in treating and preventing Alzheimer's disease requires a more detailed approach. It seems helpful to me to draw attention to the clinical studies that focus only on testosterone levels. That does not allow for a precise estimate of androgen levels. Future studies should evaluate daily androgen production. For example, a blood testosterone level of 600 ng/100 mL can correspond to pathology in men. On the other hand, a 350 ng/100 mL level can indicate nonpathological metabolism and may not require hormonal substitution. Therefore, dihydrotestosterone measurement is always essential.

The double-blind experimental setup is necessary for clinical studies. They make it possible to get a general idea of the results while eliminating subjective factors. Moreover, such studies are convenient for direct research.

But I would like to draw attention to the hormonal singularity of each person who has Alzheimer's disease. It is advisable to make a <u>detailed study of androgen</u> metabolism **in each patient**. The singular study of androgens in each person with Alzheimer's disease makes it possible to prescribe a precise and well-proportioned androgen treatment. Testosterone is not the only androgen available; for men and women, mesterolone is the right drug. Administration of a standard testosterone dose is not conducive to treating each person. Standard amounts always constitute a therapeutic approximation. The biology is singular for each patient and may imply a specific treatment with androgens or a possible singular counterindication to this treatment. Failing this, a single and standard testosterone amount can lead to undesirable effects.

A better knowledge of therapy with androgens should be part of university education. The administered doses are often too weak or too strong. To consider a standard testosterone dose for each patient is not reasonable. The doses of insulin or thyroxine required to treat diabetes or thyroid insufficiency vary from person to person. Future clinical studies and medication need a detailed analysis of androgen metabolism in people with Alzheimer's. To better understand the treatment and hormonal prevention of this disease.

The regularization of androgen metabolism is necessary from the appearance of the first symptoms of Alzheimer's disease. Upstream, the early signs of menopausal disease signal. In 2012, researchers at the

University of Tokyo and Hamamatsu University School of Medicine in Shizuoka, Japan, showed the beneficial effect of testosterone on cognitive function in mice and its inhibition of senescence in the vascular endothelial cells of the hippocampus*[15].

Destruction of nerve cells begins in the depths of the brain in the structure called the *hippocampus*. Then the destroyed cerebral tissue extends gradually into increasingly broad cerebral zones. Finally, damage to the whole brain causes death after many years of confusion and dementia. According to several scientific observations, testosterone has shown its neuroprotective effect on neuronal death for fifteen years (see the previous discussion).

In 2014, Chinese researchers studied the mechanism of β-amyloid protein toxicity on synaptic transmission† and its simultaneous effect with testosterone. Their discovery is of high importance. Researchers studied the neuronal cells of the hippocampus from rats in culture, in contact with β-amyloid proteins and testosterone.

The general effect of the β-amyloid protein‡ was to reduce synaptic transmission. The Chinese study confirmed the protective effect of testosterone on synaptic transmission in the presence of β-amyloid protein. Researchers made these discoveries in various institutions in the Republic of China [16].

---

* Hippocampus: a small cerebral convolution whose form represents the shape of a small fish of the same name. This structure is deep within the human brain. It is responsible for memory and space orientation. The nerve cells of the hippocampus can multiply in adulthood.

† A synapse is a functional zone of contact between two neurons or between a neuron and another cell (muscle cells, sensory receptors).

‡ eta-amyloid protein is a peptide consisting of forty to forty-two amino acids.

Mechanisms of cerebral lesions when the production of male hormones is insufficient	
Normal production of androgens	Insufficient production of androgens
↓	↓
Small permeable arteries	Small blocked arteries
↓	↓
Normal nervous cells Active hormonal receivers	Destroyed nervous cells Destroyed hormonal receivers
↓	↓
Normal production of myelin New ramifications of nervous fibers	Abnormal production of myelin ↓ Ruptures of nervous fibers' ramifications ↓ Accumulation of proteins β-amyloid ↓ Autoimmunity reactions
Vascularization is typical in the whole brain. Receivers of androgens are activated in the whole brain.	In the beginning, vascularization is defective in the profound parts of the brain and then in its totality. Receivers of androgens are not activated anymore in cerebral territories.
↓	↓
Normal brain	Dementias

The doctor confronted with Alzheimer's disease has few means of treatment because the destruction of nerve cells is always definitive. Therefore, treatment of Alzheimer's disease is initially preventive. It is necessary to act from the beginning of the illness, such as when one forgets unceasingly where the keys are. Therapy with androgens at the beginning of Alzheimer's disease would represent significant progress because the condition would likely stop advancing at this stage. That would make it possible to avoid losing the keys all the time after age forty and to avoid developing insanity after that. This approach would also enable many of the diseases of ageing described in this book to be prevented. Not counting the fundamental impact of testosterone on the maintenance of cerebral artery patency, can one neglect the regenerating effect of male hormones on the ramifications of the brain's nerve cells?

In short, testosterone production decreases with age in men and women. Androgens act through several well-identified mechanisms. Male hormones have the following functions:

- Stimulate growth, ramification, and insulation of nervous fibers
- Prevent cerebral arteries from being affected by sclerosis
- Avoid the production of β-amyloid protein and its consequent deposition in the brain
- Prevention of Alzheimer's disease from the appearance of the first symptoms and even before, when the production of male hormones is insufficient

Simple testosterone levels are insufficient to establish the diagnosis. A detailed study of androgen production is essential in each person (man or woman) who has Alzheimer's disease. Biochemical detection of deficits and their therapeutic correction are quite important, particularly at the beginning of the disease. Treatment of androgen deficits is safe (chapter 33). Clinical and biological studies conducted in this direction will quickly give positive results

Summary

Major pharmaceutical companies have abandoned research on molecules that did not provide any effects on Alzheimer's disease. The pharmaceutical problem is that the industry is interested only in the final phase of the illness, whereas this treatment began decades earlier.

Arteriosclerosis prevention and the diminution of abnormal amyloid protein production prevent Alzheimer's disease. The prevention starts by regulating androgens with mesterolone in men and women after forty.

Alzheimer's disease is a global disaster that can affect anyone. Interesting studies have indicated testosterone and Alzheimer's disease [1–16]. Their results will be better understood through new research that considers the following:

- Studies generally look at blood testosterone levels without regard to blood dihydrotestosterone levels.

- At the same time, dihydrotestosterone is a significant source of androgen hormone production.

- Hormonal studies are generally concerned only with blood testosterone levels. Not with the hormone's total and daily production of its precursors and metabolites.

- Studies on sex hormones that do not consider dihydrotestosterone and testosterone production and all androgen precursors and metabolites are therefore incomplete and challenging to interpret—even unusable.

- It seems to me that it is consequently logical to carry out urgently those new studies. There is no reason to wait.

30
Stroke

A stroke is a sudden neurological deficit of vascular origin caused by infarction or hemorrhage of the brain. Fifteen percent of strokes are hemorrhagic, generally causing hemiplegia. Signs vary depending on the localization of the cerebral lesion. This kind of stroke usually results from sudden arterial hypertension, which has produced a rupture of a blood vessel wall. This incident is sometimes the result of an inadequately adjusted anticoagulant treatment. Eighty percent of strokes are ischemic. Diabetes and hypertension are the principal causes because these diseases lead to a thickening of the walls of small cerebral arteries until their occlusion. The lack of oxygen causes the death of the nerve cells. The probability of having an ischemic stroke increases with age.

Prevalence

In the United States, there are 795,000 strokes each year, of which 610,000 represent a first brain attack, and 185,000 cases constitute relapses. A person has an attack every forty seconds [1].

According to the World Health Organization (WHO), Strokes are a pandemic. An increased incidence will lead from 16 million in 2005 to 23 million in 2030. In addition, mortality from stroke will increase from 5.7 to 12 million in the same period [2].

Symptoms

Apparent symptoms are the loss of mobility of an arm or a leg, deviation of the mouth, and paralysis of half of the body. Other symptoms, such as difficulty expressing oneself or eye troubles, are alarming.

In 2011, stroke was the twentieth-leading cause of death in the United States. A person dies of a stroke every four minutes [1].

Twenty to 30 per cent of patients with strokes die in the first three months, 45 per cent die in six months, and 70 per cent die in five years.

The cost of strokes in the United States reaches $34 billion annually [3], including medical benefits, drugs, and work incapacities. In Canada, the annual cost of strokes is $3.6 billion.

Ischemic stroke does not occur by chance. It is generally the consequence of the obstruction of a cerebral artery by a narrowing of its diameter or by a clot, which destroys cerebral tissue. Stroke caused by ageing results from the degradation of the organism:

- Fatty untreated diabetes (chapter 10)
- Triglycerides and cholesterol excess (chapter 11)
- Atheroma (chapter 11)
- Excess weight and obesity (chapter 12)
- Arterial rigidity or Arteriosclerosis (chapter 14)
- Anemia (chapter 15)
- Thick blood (chapter 16)
- Untreated hypertension (chapter 17)
- Coronary disease and myocardial infarction (chapter 18)
- Degeneration of connective tissue (chapter 19)
- Deterioration of nervous system (chapter 29)

In other words, a man of age seventy who measures 1.80 meters in height, weighs 160 pounds, has a healthy blood pressure of 12/8, and has a cholesterol level of 150 mg/100 mL of plasma has little chance of having a stroke in the immediate future. In contrast, a man of seventy who measures 1.80 meters in height, weighs 250 pounds, has a blood pressure of 16/10, and has a cholesterol level of 260 mg/100 mL of plasma is likely to have a stroke or a heart attack in the immediate future.

A stroke is a medical emergency that requires immediate action and medical care. The speed with which the stroke victim arrives at a hospital offering specialized services for acute stroke determines the chance of survival with few or no incapacities. Unfortunately, the public generally ignores the characteristics of a stroke and the importance of detecting, in time, the risk factor preceding the stroke: hypertension.

Stroke and Dementia

Vascular dementia is a disorder caused by multiple minor cerebral vascular incidents in the brain that generate a variety of cognitive symptoms, including memory disorders.

Strokes constitute the first cause of a physical handicap acquired in adults and the second cause of dementia after Alzheimer's.

Part IV

Revitalize your Body

*Long desires
of spring days
will not be forgotten
when autumn comes
in the heart of men.*

—*SHUISHÛ,*
around the year 1000

31

The Anti-Ageing Hormone

There are phenomena whose causes and symptoms are apparent. For example, a drop in blood pressure caused by external bleeding, with its spectacular manifestation, is understood more quickly because it is simple: trauma. However, if the cause is internal bleeding, it is a little more complicated; it is necessary to identify the organ responsible for the bleeding. Immediate treatment consists of a blood transfusion, but the bleeding should be stopped simultaneously through wound closure and possible removal of the diseased organ.

A brief look back in time will show how a disease can persist for centuries without people knowing it. In the case of this disease, billions of human beings died prematurely without knowing why.

Before the Second World War, infectious diseases still caused devastation in the West. However, archaeological discoveries showed that this specific disease has existed since antiquity. The remains of bodies showed inflammatory tumours in all organs. Tubercular lesions were also found in Egyptian mummies.

Aristotle had already recognised the contagiousness of the disease, and Hippocrates, noting the extreme exhaustion of the patients, had given the disease the name phthisis.

The bloody sputum of the Lady to the Camellias (*La Dame aux camélias*) remained famous and was a tragedy of ignorance.

In 1819, Laennec, an exceptional doctor, recognised the uniqueness of the disease. In his treatise on the stethoscope, he affirmed that all tubercular lesions from the lung transformed into a huge abscess and then destroyed the kidneys. Moreover, the deformed bones producing hunchbacks resulted from the same disease.

For more than fifty years, this theory was the object of controversy; most doctors could not see the relationship between hunchbacks and bloody sputum. The great outdoors and rest were the only treatments. The cause of the disease was unknown. Deaths amounted to millions.

In 1882, Koch described the bacillus responsible for the tubercular lesions. The cause of the disease was finally found, but people didn't die less because of it. It was necessary to find the remedy and to wait sixty-two more years. In 1944, Waksman discovered streptomycin. Consequently, tuberculosis would be overcome. But it was also necessary to have the antibiotic. One can still die of tuberculosis in 2017 in the Third World due to a lack of information and money.

Closer to our time, AIDS was very quickly identified in a few years despite the diversity of its symptoms: lung infection, cerebral abscesses, and skin cancer, known as Kaposi disease. Thanks to the power of scientific research, Luc Montagnier and his team quickly identified the cause of this condition by isolating the responsible virus. Several drugs have already knocked back the disease. AZT and now quadruple therapy delayed the virus's progression. The interferons cured certain Kaposi cancers. Knowledge of this pathology continues to advance, and one can hope for its control in years to come, thereby ending this plague of the twentieth century.

A disaster just as frightening threatens humanity. It exists everywhere and causes devastation: ageing diseases. They are omnipresent and presented in such different forms that they do not seem to have any relationship. And yet, why, when men get old, is there suddenly this blow one day that unrelentingly leads them toward decrepitude, passing the second half of their lives with disease and suffering? Why are they generally in good health before forty? If a basic principle explains good health, that is what is lacking when the body begins to degrade. Some will say it is genetic, but everything is genetic. Therefore, it is not a sufficient explanation. If it is genetic, the information must be translated as meaning something.

And what if ageing starts entirely only with the incapacity to secrete the hormone of life: testosterone?

From 1945 to now, medicine has triumphed in many fields thanks to a whole panoply of increasingly sophisticated drugs and techniques. As a result, the man's life expectancy in developed Western countries, which was 54 at the beginning of the twentieth century, has risen to 81.2 years today, in the country where men live longest: Iceland.

The median age progresses, keeping people barely alive, isolated in their tiny rooms, armchairs, or nailed onto the bed.

The disease can be defeated only when the cause is defined and the remedy found.

And what if the cause of sexual ageing is the same as that which starts general ageing?

The testicles produce between seven and ten milligrams of testosterone daily. This quantity is distributed throughout the organism and acts locally, with amounts measured in picograms (thousandths of a billionth gram).

The genitals use only one small part of this production. The most significant quantity of secreted testosterone is used by all organs of the human body, which need some to maintain and regenerate their protein structures, without which no life is possible.

Consequently, seven to ten thousand billionths of a gram is necessary daily to make the organism function and maintain the organs in a good state.

This fact explains many diseases that occur after age forty. They appear according to each individual's unique biology and worsen unrelentingly over time.

The following disorders appear in the man with an androgenic disease of andropause; general weaknesses are also common.

Sexual Ageing

- Impotence
- Ejaculation disorders
- Prostate problems

General Diseases of Ageing

- Excess weight
- Obesity
- Intestinal distension
- Osteoarthritis (shoulder, knee, hip, spinal column)
- Brittleness of the articular ligaments
- Osteoporosis (osseous brittleness, fractures)
- Muscular brittleness
- Hypertension
- Angina pectoris
- Myocardial infarction
- Arteriosclerosis
- Varicose veins
- Hemorrhoids
- Varicose ulcers
- Gangrene
- Anemia
- Thick blood
- Arterial or venous thrombosis
- A rise in blood cholesterol (especially bad cholesterol)
- The increase in blood triglycerides

- Diabetes
- Wrinkles
- Inadequate filtration of the kidneys and uremia
- Immunizing deficit, predisposing to cancers
- Vision trouble
- Hearing disorders
- Loose teeth
- Depression, the wrong image of oneself, irritability, melancholy, suicidal tendency, incapacity to act
- Migraine headaches
- Inability to react to stress

At first sight, these numerous diseases and symptoms do not appear to be related. Therefore, attempting to find their link may seem deceptive.

A first reflection is essential: Do these symptoms, groups of signs, or diseases exist? The answer is yes. Anyone can observe that.

Then, are these gathered phenomena the expression of ageing? The answer is yes. Let us consider older men. They present these apparent disorders.

The third point is essential to this reflection. A common link connects all these phenomena: they can be caused in whole or in part by a lack of male hormones. It is a fact shown by many scientific studies published over many years. Continuation of the reasoning comes logically. If the hormone is missing, why not give it to those who show a decrease in androgen production?

But does this hormone exist in the form of drugs? The answer is, yet again, yes. Testosterone has been available since 1936 in the form of intramuscular injections.

We have the symptoms, the disease, and the antidote. We should not be losing a moment.

The phenomena of ageing appear successively. First, they appear as symptoms treated by traditional medicine. But each degenerative event can trigger others, which can cause still other symptoms.

It is like a Russian doll, where each doll hides a smaller one, and so on. One can imagine a similar system where one puppet would be replaced by a chicken and another by an egg. Each chicken would hide a smaller egg, which, in turn, would conceal a smaller chicken. One cannot escape the fundamental questions: Where does the chicken come from, and where does the egg originate? Regarding ageing diseases, the problem becomes more complicated. The chickens and the eggs are different colors. It follows a seemingly inextricable tangle, a labyrinth from which it can only leave thanks to a guiding thread (*le fil d'Ariane*). This thread is the male hormone.

Excess weight and obesity involve the overloading of bones and joint articulations, which wear more quickly, accelerating the appearance of osteoarthritis. At the same time, the body mass needs more blood flow, and the blood pressure rises automatically. I will mention just three complications with this example for ease of presentation. First, the overload of the organism causes mechanical wear of joint articulations and an increase in blood pressure. Second, a lack of male hormones leads to increased fat accumulation and excess weight. Third, the walls of the arteries become rigid from a lack of male hormones, thus causing hypertension that worsens with overweight.

The same phenomenon occurs in fragile joint articulations. Deprived of male hormones, they crush more easily when there is an overload. Therefore, to prevent degeneration and maintain the human body's good health, it is necessary to address pathological factors simultaneously.

Mesterolone is the right anti-ageing hormone for technical reasons, as we will see later (chapter 33).

32

Control your Ageing

Sexual ageing and the general ageing of the human body are syndromes. Treating a body without considering its condition is not enough, because in this case, there is no solution. The general condition of the human body must be the object of individual attention.

Beyond age forty, the body is often more destroyed than we think. The degenerative transformations are already apparent to the observer who can see (it is enough to open one's eyes). If you are over forty, don't you believe you are sick? Look attentively at yourself naked in a mirror. Observe your face, chest, belly, profile, arms, and legs. Compare this image with one of your photographs in a swimsuit between twenty and twenty-five. The differences are due to ageing.

Is your face the same one? Do you recognize yourself? Do you accept the pasted-on look, its solidified features, inexpressive mimicry, and sad glance?

Does your well-developed thorax allow full or reduced breathing? Does it allow only weak, superficial breathing? Are you the same size as you were at twenty-five?

Does your belly resemble a stratospheric balloon more and more? Are your buttocks made of fat or muscles? What became of your arms and your legs?

What is the state of your skin? Did you lose your pilosity? Are your nails hard or breakable? Are your breasts prominent? Did you get shorter by one or several centimeters? Are your shoulders arched? Is your back aligned?

Now go to the silhouettes of the regressive man (figure 13, page 116). At age twenty-five, the silhouette represents the man at the peak of his development. The profiles at 30, 40, and 55 years of age are all degenerative. Locate your silhouette. Do not be afraid. Even if you correspond to the drawing of fifty-five years, you can go the opposite way, successively passing by the silhouettes of forty and thirty years. In the best case, while working on yourself, you will reach the age of twenty-five.

The ideal is to react quickly and not enter the extreme forms of degeneration.

Visible damage outside is the expression of devastation inside the body, in all organs, including the brain.

The damage caused by a lack of rest, immobility, self-destruction by tobacco use, and unhealthy food is considerable. Control of these harmful factors is essential and constitutes a precondition to the biochemical control of the body after age forty. Smokers, the sedentary or overly stressed, alcoholics, and the obese have short lives.

Early sexual problems, depression, and micturition problems lead many men to go for consultations. They hope for a miracle cure to solve all their problems. But doctors are not always aware that male hormones can be missing in men.

Furthermore, biologically maintaining and prolonging an older body's existence is unrealizable without a healthy lifestyle. Therefore, at the risk of upsetting some candidates for longevity, I tell them from the start: do not smoke, arrange your working time, and exercise.

People are what they eat and what they drink. At one level, drinking and eating involve something pleasant and friendly. However, in terms of longevity, food is essential; alcohol and fat make a mess of male hormones.

Chronic alcoholism gradually destroys the liver; patients with cirrhosis have perturbed sex hormones. In addition, the disease of alcoholism destroys the integrity of the nervous system and the testicles. Under these conditions, alcoholics are bad candidates for hormonal replacement therapy.

Excess fat is also damaging—a more massive silhouette results from the fatty degeneration of the body. The overload starts with the first extra pound. It is common to note excesses of twenty to forty pounds and more. Did you calculate your body mass index (BMI) on this subject? (If not, see chapter 12.)

Fat can collect and neutralize male hormones. Therefore, to ensure effective hormonal treatment, it is necessary to eliminate unnecessary fat at all costs by controlling your diet. If you have a weight problem, learn the energy value of food and the various dietetic methods by consulting the many books covering this issue. If necessary, do not hesitate to consult your doctor. The goal is to reach the weight you were between twenty and twenty-five years old (if you did not have a weight problem).

A simple blood test is sometimes enough to diagnose hormonal insufficiency. However, a complete study of hormonal production is often necessary. Levels of sex hormones at a given time provide the ideal hormonal profile in men from age twenty to twenty-five, not presenting any organic or degenerative sexual problem. These biological conditions are necessary to restore one's youth as much as possible.

33

Hormonal Treatment

Birth of the Concept

At the beginning of the 1970s, I realized that the hormonal aspect of sexual disorders was unknown. I had just obtained my *agrégation in urology**.

Because impotent men were considered "psychopaths," university education about this pathology was nonexistent. But I considered the situation because there were numerous complaints in similar terms about the same symptoms or identical symptom groups. It was one of two things: either the hundreds of patients who complained about impotence were insane, and the doctor who diagnosed psychopathy was right, or the patients were correct, and it was the doctor who was entirely off. I took the patients' side and decided to study the problem from a hormonal perspective, mainly because hormone levels could be easily measured by 1974. I quickly realized that older men's male hormone levels were decreased, initially causing medically reversible impotence or mechanical impotence due to arteriosclerosis when the hormonal deficit had caused its destructive effects. So, I started prescribing hormones in quantity, with increasingly convincing results. And I placed penile implants surgically in impotent patients with blocked arteries, with highly encouraging results.

I was teaching at Brussels University, covering the Andrology part of the Urology course. Unfortunately, the urology professor had been ill

---

* In Europe, for some disciplines of higher education, such as urology, there is an *agrégation* for the professorship positions called *agrégation de l'enseignement supérieur*.

for a long time, so I drew up urology examinations for the third-year medical students.

The hospital director where I worked decided to create a university department specializing in andrology, parallel to the urology department. As in any pyramidal structure, the chief watched over the service, ensuring he did not lose power. Depending on the university, the hospital, and the "chief," a commission was arranged with his old friends, sitting behind closed doors, to file a scientific lawsuit against me. What could be better than instituting a special court to bar me at all costs? They declared me insane because I treated and operated on impotence, whereas everyone knew it was a mental disease. Deemed "crazy," I joined the rows of demented patients (one has the doctor one deserves). Determined to fight to clear up andropause problems, I decided to leave the hospital.

Two years later, after a stormy debate over whether a young chief could cohabit with an old boss, the university's board of directors granted my resignation with some hesitation. My career as an associate professor was thus cut short after such a promising beginning!

Meanwhile, I had created, in 1974, a private medical center specializing in andrology, which increasingly received more patients. This private clinic specializing in sexual pathology was probably one of the first, if not the first, in Europe. In addition, I had the honor to receive many doctors who had been my medical professors and professors at other universities, whose condition necessitated andrological surgery, specific hormonal treatment with androgens, or both.

The patients began to flow into my private clinic. It quickly became evident that organic impotence was part of a whole—sexual ageing being the consequence of a hormonal insufficiency that caused disorders not only of erection but also of ejaculation and prostate diseases.

Treatment of benign prostate hypertrophy and of organic impotence reached three great stages thanks to the benefits of hormonal replacement therapy:

In the 1960s, men presenting a prostatic disorder were operated on with an open belly, and the surgery of organic impotence did not exist.

In the 1970s, men with a prostatic disease requiring surgery underwent a more delicate operation, the endoscopic prostate resection, made through natural ways. Organic impotence was treated systematically by penile silicone implants.

For a few years, urologists have used lasers in an endoscopic way to destroy the tissue of the sick prostate.

Today, the same prostatic disorders are controlled by hormonal replacement therapy, delaying or avoiding prostate surgery for several years. Impotence due to the androgenic disease of andropause responds to hormonal treatment in 90 percent of cases. The operation for organic impotence has more limited indications.

During the 1970s, I realized that the patients treated with hormones for their sexual ageing often said, "I climb better," or "I don't have knee pain anymore." Others said, "I win again when playing tennis," "My joint pains disappeared," "I regained my memory," and "I am not depressed anymore." At the same time, I noted improvements in blood sugar, cholesterol, and other blood parameters. Sexual and general ageing seemed linked by a common cause: insufficient sex hormone secretion. They were guide threads that explained the degeneration from the androgenic disease of andropause.

By consulting the world's medical literature, one can note that many researchers work separately on the beneficial properties of testosterone in all fields. Their high-quality work is essential. Their synthesis enabled me to confirm what the clinical study suggests: sexual ageing and the general ageing of the human body regress with the administration of male hormones.

At What Age to Begin the Treatment?

The sexual and general ageing signs caused by low male hormone levels indicate hormonal replacement treatment. It must be undertaken from the first symptoms. When those appear, hormonal insufficiency exists for many months or many years. To eliminate the most regressive phenomena, their appearance should be prevented. It is too late to act when sclerosis is installed. Hormonal treatment can begin at any age to recover what can be improved and avoid further degeneration. The ideal would be to prevent ageing from the appearance of the first clinical symptom, and even before. An annual clinical and biological checkup should be carried out systematically from the age of forty to prevent hormonal insufficiency.

Are Androgens the Cause of Prostate Cancer?

Prostate cancer caused by androgens was never shown in man; on the contrary, however, the rumour existed, and it has thick skin. If you meet someone who affirms this untruth, ask him for any proof. He will not be able to give it to you; it does not exist. Many recent publications prove that hormone replacement therapy with androgens is safe, which is not part of this book. Significant progress will be made in the future.

It is possible to consult the world's medical literature online. However, prostatic cancer in men caused by the administration of male hormones is not described.

At the time of puberty, male hormones invade the body massively. If testosterone is carcinogenic, teenagers should develop many cancers. However, it is not the case.

Since the introduction of androgens into therapeutic use (the traditional indications are numerous: treatment of anemias, leukemia, great testicular insufficiencies, and so on), the mortality caused by prostate cancer has not increased statistically. I sought to know the importance of the pharmaceutical industry's annual production of male hormones. It is impossible to know—it is an industrial secret.

Cancer. Hormone. Prostate. Each one of these words can arouse strong passions. Cancer is not well understood. A minimum of biochemical and biological knowledge is necessary to conceive the hormone. Most men do not know the structure and the function of the prostate. The mixture of these three concepts often starts irrational reactions. Calmly let us see the facts.

One cannot prevent oneself from comparing the increase in the frequency of prostate cancer beyond age fifty with the progressive lowering of male hormone secretion. But unfortunately, the two phenomena follow opposite curves and progress with age.

In a man with an androgenic disease of andropause, the lack of male hormones causes an imbalance in favor of corticoid hormones. As a result, the destruction of malignant cells is compromised, and, generally, cancer develops more quickly.

The seventy-year-old men who develop prostate cancer are statistically deprived of male hormones in the male population. Consequently, in a man with an androgenic disease of andropause, the well-proportioned hormonal treatment with male hormones would prevent prostate cancer.

In 1996, a scientific study by the James Buchanan Brady Urological Institute, The Johns Hopkins University School of Medicine, Baltimore Maryland, showed the beneficial effects of androgens on the prostate of rats, as assessed by telomere analysis* and telomerase†enzyme activity in seminal vesicles and prostate glands.

The conclusions are as follows [1]:

- The normal glands of the ventral prostate and rat seminal vesicles do not show telomerase activity.
- Telomerase activity appears when these glands degenerate following castration.
- On the contrary, telomerase activity disappears when these glands regenerate under the influence of testosterone.
- It is the first living model to demonstrate telomerase regulation.

The biological mechanism is probably the same one in man.

This biological study confirms in rats what my rigorous clinical observation of man has indicated for decades: androgens are necessary to maintain healthy prostate structures by preventing the anarchistic cells' multiplication [2].

Not all mechanisms of telomere shortening are understood, but oxidative stress from local inflammation might accelerate prostatic telomere loss [3].

---

* Telomeres: noncoding sequence of DNA at the end of eukaryotic chromosomes. The telomeres shorten with each cell division and are a signal of cellular senescence (cell ageing).
Telomerase: an enzyme whose function is to maintain the length of the telomeres, thus allowing the unlimited division of the cell. This enzyme is associated with the concept of cancer cell immortality.

Which Hormones to Take for Androgenic Disease?

Insanity is doing the same thing repeatedly and expecting a different result.

Albert Einstein

In recent years, more than 25,000 lawsuits have been filed against manufacturers of testosterone products due to side effects that were life-threatening or fatal. Most complaints were settled. Low-T is not a diagnosis but is a marketing term coined to describe symptoms such as fatigue, low sex drive, and loss of muscle tone. These men may have suffered severe complications due to testosterone replacement therapy.

When considering all available routes of delivery, concentrations, and branded or generic choices, there are currently over 30 testosterone preparations to consider.

ThoseTestosterone products can cause serious side effects:

- Blood clots
- Myocardial infarction or heart attack
- Cerebrovascular accident or stroke
- Pulmonary embolism
- Deep vein thrombosis
- Venous thromboembolism
- Death

> **Testosterone products** used to mistakenly treat low testosterone syndrome in the elderly are administered intramuscularly, orally, or percutaneously with a gel.
>
> **These products are not the treatment of the androgenic disease.**

> Notwithstanding claims regarding those products, the drug/medical device remains approved by the U.S. FDA for treatment of hypogonadism **only.**

Which Hormones to Take?

Androgens are "classically" used to treat hypogonadism. Low testosterone syndrome in older people does not indicate a need for testosterone supplementation. Those androgens can be managed through intramuscular, oral, or percutaneous methods. They **are not the treatment for the androgenic disease of andropause** [21,24].

The treatment for the androgenic disease of andropause is mesterolone, an effective and non-toxic molecule.

> **Mesterolone has been available since 1966 and is the leading hormone to treat the androgenic disease of andropause**.

Mesterolone has the same molecular structure as dihydrotestosterone. It is missing in the first stage of androgenic andropause disease—the sexual ageing. It also has molecular properties similar to those of testosterone, which decrease over time. So, it is possible to treat the two stages of the androgenic disease of andropause safely and on time. This hormone is available as 25-milligram tablets. It would be interesting to have 10-milligram tablets. The maximum concentration of mesterolone in the blood is reached at the third hour after taking it and decreases thereafter. The daily amount is generally divided into two: morning and midday, or morning and evening. Mesterolone is an inexpensive generic drug marketed under the brand names Provibol®, Provironum®, and Proviron®, as well as mesterolone. Mesterolone is **not transformed into female hormones** (estradiol). Instead, it is converted by the liver (which removes its methyl radical) into dihydrotestosterone, a **natural hormone**. It is also mesterolone that is necessary, but at lower doses, to prevent and cure urinary problems, pain during intercourse, and some diseases of ageing in women. This topic was presented at the SEMAL congress in Madrid in October 2015 [4].

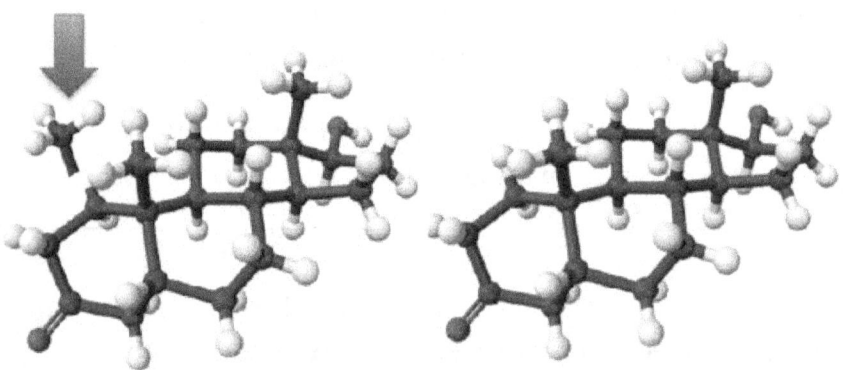

Mesterolone　　　　　Dihydrotestosterone

> Androgenic andropause disease begins forty years before the total collapse of testosterone and dihydrotestosterone production. Then it is too late to prevent the diseases of ageing that have developed during those forty years.

Any hormonal treatment is to be performed under medical supervision. The treatment of androgenic disease of andropause or menopause is not testosterone but **mesterolone. This molecule has testosterone and dihydrotestosterone properties**. Mesterolone is used, preferably for technical reasons [5-6-7].

Contraindications - Warning

The lack of indication is the first contraindication. It is useless to take male hormones when treatment is not necessary. The inability to understand the effects of hormones and the intellectual failure to control food are contraindications to hormone replacement therapy. Testosterone treatments are available as gels, creams, patches, pills, tablets, and injections. There are class actions against pharmaceutical companies that market these products at doses that might be inappropriate in the US. The androgenic disease of andropause is unknown, and, therefore, its treatment is unknown. Testosterone gel in large quantities is anything. Class actions in the US are due to the **misuse of testosterone**. Androgenic diseases of andropause or menopause are not teached in universities.

Each patient requires a unique treatment. For example, one milligram of testosterone is not 10 milligrams. Does each doctor prescribe a standard dose of fifty insulin units to each diabetic patient?

Renal, cardiac, and severe hepatic insufficiency cause serious disorders for which it is advisable to consider the hormonal effects. The state of aggressiveness accentuated by male hormones contraindicates their employment. Adenoma and prostate cancer need specific treatment (chapter 9).

Harmful Side Effects

Excess weight, water retention, and salt retention are consequences of mismanaged hormonal treatment. The overdose of hormones primarily causes these pernicious effects. Signs of overdose disappear after the suspension of excessive hormonal therapy. Reduced and adapted quantities can be prescribed without causing the same perverse effects. The taking of male hormones increases protein synthesis. If, at the same time, the food is not controlled, excess weight is inevitable. Treating male hormones requires comprehending their effects and reflecting on oneself, which imposes nutritional control. Without any thought, the man treated with male hormones evolves as a calf does under hormonal influence. The calf does not think. It eats. Thanks to anabolic hormones, it consumes more. As a result, it weighs more—to the greatest happiness of the adulterated meat merchants. Thanks to nutrition knowledge, taking hormones and losing weight are possible. Liver overload can occur when there is an overdose or an incapacity to control food intake. However, a synthetic hormone can be poorly tolerated by the liver: 17-alpha-methyltestosterone, which must be avoided.

On the other hand, mesterolone's hepatic tolerance is remarkable. Unfortunately, mesterolone, a safe hormone sold worldwide, is unavailable in the US for mysterious reasons. At the same time, 17 alpha-methyl testosterone, which must be avoided because of its side effects, is marketed in the US.

Once the hormonal balance is reached, monitoring the hormonal profile and maintenance treatment are performed annually. The liver's function is controlled simultaneously. Since the beginning of my clinical experience, I have not encountered a single case of hepatic intolerance. On the contrary, some cases of hepatic insufficiency improved with male hormones, which have a regenerative effect on hepatic cells.

Doping

Doping has been a topic of discussion in sporting magazines for many years. The high-level athletes increase their muscular mass, and consequently their performances, by absorbing anabolic drugs, among which testosterone or its derivatives occupy a place of choice.

Young athletes generally have a normal secretion of male hormones. Consequently, they do not have any medical reason to absorb these drugs. They can naturally produce higher levels of male hormones than their elders, who cannot win at the Olympic Games after age forty. As a result, natural energy decreases over the years.

The challenges are considerable; athletes do not hesitate to infringe on the rules of the sport and absorb anything. Swallowing the tablets with frenzy, they are doped temporarily for transitory successes, endangering their health. Moreover, hormones' useless, awkward, and excessive absorption can cause harmful side effects.

Some also recently proposed the administration of high testosterone amounts to cause the temporary sterility of young men by blocking the formation of spermatozoa in the testicles. This kind of contraception can have the same fatal consequences as doping. The public and even doctors amalgamate doping problems and the therapeutic use of male hormones. With unreasoned fears, they say that hormones are harmful. Sex hormones are necessary for life. It is their perverse use that is harmful.

Treatment of the Andropause Androgenic Disease

It must be undertaken with understanding to avoid disappointment [8] from the androgen replacement treatment. Insulin is not prescribed blindly. It is the same with androgens.
Each man is singular. His biology varies during ageing. Therefore, hormonal analyses are particularly important throughout life and in

relation to treatments. Hormone treatment must always be under a doctor's supervision.

The treatment depends on the clinical situation at a given time and the doctor's experience.

The amounts to be managed are particularly delicate in older men still secreting a certain quantity of male hormones. Indeed, one does not suffer from hypogonadism at once. The reduction in the production of male hormones is progressive, and the hormonal replacement should be neither insufficient nor excessive.

If the degradation of sexual organs is not too advanced, the treatment often produces spectacular effects. The erection becomes valid again. Urination disorders improve. At the same time, all structures of the organism regenerate.

An overdose appears immediately through excessive nervousness. It is enough to reduce the amount to find the correct quantity. The treatment continues with daily administration of an optimal hormonal dose.

The treatment is given by mouth, generally divided into two doses throughout the day.

The more surprising effect of the male hormone maintenance treatment is to prevent sexual ageing and delay the general ageing of the human body. It is a long-term, primarily preventive effect that requires reflection. The treatment must be continued for life.

Monitoring the Treatment

The blood levels of testosterone and dihydrotestosterone are already significant. But global androgen metabolism should be analysed if necessary. In all cases, under the control of a doctor, it is required:

- To maintain blood pressure close to 12/8, and a pulse of 72.
- Avoid excessive weight gain (fat or muscle) by controlling your food intake.

- Follow the evolution of the number of red and white blood cells.
- Control in the blood: glucose, cholesterol, triglycerides (fats).
- Control blood fluidity (antithrombin) and proteins.
- Total bilirubin (liver indicator).

In addition to the clinical examination, all these data determine the androgen hormone and dose.

Is Long-Term Treatment with Androgens without Danger?

For more than forty years, doctors who prescribed continuous therapy with androgens have always affirmed the safety of the treatment for **hypogonadism.**

For over thirty years, Jens Møeller prescribed testosterone to treat cardiovascular diseases [9]. However, he never noted the appearance of prostate cancer under treatment.

Since 1974, I have prescribed **mesterolone for the androgenic disease of andropause.** Since then, I have never seen the appearance of invading prostate cancer in more than a thousand men following continuous hormone therapy, their prostates being checked clinically and biologically every year. Although many doctors followed this therapeutic method, none told me of any incident. The hormonal treatment in men with an androgenic disease of andropause stabilizes the prostatic tissues. As a result, urination remains stable, thus delaying or avoiding the need for surgery. In addition, **mesterolone** is necessary to normalize prostate structures [2]. Mesterolone is not testosterone but methylated dihydrotestosterone in C1 (Carbon 1). I described mesterolone use in detail in 2025 in *Androgenic Disease in Men* [16].

For seventy-two months, androgen therapy was done in thirty-five men with **hypogonadism**. Doses were from eighty to two hundred milligrams of testosterone undecanoate daily. Among the treated men, eight were between fifty and sixty-two years old. This interesting study, about hypogonadism treatment published in 1986 by Gooren L.J.D., showed for six years the perfect harmlessness of treatment with testosterone undecanoate [11].

In 2012, M. R. Feneley of the Institute of Urology and Nephrology, University Hospital College, London, and M. Carruthers from the Center for Men's Health, London, published a study relating to 1,365 men from twenty-eight to eighty-seven years old (average fifty-five) who had presented a deficiency in androgens. The monitoring dates back twenty years. The authors conclude that the treatment with testosterone under regular monitoring of the prostate can be more secure than any alternative without control. The data were compared across four androgen preparations: testosterone pellet implants, Restandol, Testogel, and mesterolone [12].

In 2012, *The Journal of Clinical Endocrinology and Metabolism* published the first study showing that untreated men having low testosterone levels (less than 250 nanograms per hundred milliliters of plasma) have a higher mortality rate than men treated with testosterone [13].

Various medical centers carried out this study for veterans in the United States (Veterans Affairs, Puget Sound Health Care System; Epidemiologic Research and Information Center GOES; GOES Geriatric Research, Education, and Clinic Center; Departments of Psychiatry and Behavioral Sciences, Epidemiology, Medicine, University of Washington, and Group Health Research Institute Group Health Cooperative, Seattle, Washington). The results relate to a cohort of 1,031 men having low testosterone rates between 2001 and 2005. They were divided into two groups.

The first group (median age 60.9) included 398 men treated with testosterone intramuscularly or with patches or cutaneous gel. Their mortality amounted to 10.3 percent throughout the study.

The second group (median age 62.8) included 633 untreated men. Their mortality amounted to 20.7 percent throughout the study, doubling the percentage of death by two.

These results show that replacement therapy with androgens significantly decreases the mortality of men having a significant deficiency (hypogonadism) of male hormones (the percentage of death is lowered by 50 percent in four years).

The authors concluded that *"these results should be interpreted cautiously because residual confounding may still be a source of bias. In addition, large, randomized clinical trials are needed to better characterize the health effects of testosterone treatment in older men with low testosterone levels"* [13].

The authors of this study are justifiably cautious. Low testosterone is not a disease; it's a biological sign. It's also surprising that the vast majority, if not all, of clinical studies on testosterone fail to mention the level of dihydrotestosterone (the natural sex hormone), which is linked to the production of testosterone, its precursor.

Sexual ageing precedes and heralds the diseases of ageing [14-15]. The androgenic disease in men causes these ageing phenomena [16].

The worst confusion is to ignore the androgenic disease of andropause prescribing the wrong treatment for this condition, i.e., testosterone.

Life expectancy can be improved when the treatment is undertaken at the beginning of an androgenic disease of andropause (chapter 4), twenty or thirty years before its final stage.

Why do the vast majority of people die before the age of 85?

The majority of people die before the age of 85 because they did not follow preventive treatment for androgenic disease starting at age 40. This universal untreated disease causes or aggravates age-related diseases known as heart disease, arteriosclerosis, metabolic diseases, fatty diabetes, rheumatic diseases, and fibrosis, such as Dupuytren's disease, Parkinson's disease, and Alzheimer's disease (Figure 24).

Consequently, a life expectancy limited to 85 years corresponds to the final stage of all these diseases.

Can prevention with mestérolone begin after the age of forty?

The transformation of normal body structures into abnormal pathological structures occurs gradually and continuously after the age of 40. Therefore, starting prevention at around 50 or 60 years of age will be done on an already partially dilapidated body. However, it is still possible to halt certain degenerative processes, thereby preventing their progression.

Is there an example of the long-term results of preventing age-related diseases with mesterolone?

My oldest patient is 85 years old and has been undergoing rigorous treatment for 47 years. To date, he has normal hematological test results, blood sugar levels of 100 mg/mL, normal cholesterol and triglyceride levels, and a PSA level of 2 ng/mL. He has a blood pressure of 11/7, a heart rate of 72, and no cardiovascular, fibrotic, or rheumatic disease. This is a favorable situation for treating possible cancer, which becomes more common with age.

Practical Matters

The Doctor

Any doctor is confronted with the androgenic disease of andropause. Particularly in an older general population over age forty, with its cardiovascular consequences, cerebral problems, and so on (see part III of this book). Consultation with the family doctor often concludes with the prescription of a cholesterol-lowering medication for cardiovascular disease, an anti-inflammatory drug for osteoarthritis, and antidepressant medication in cases of depression. These traditional treatments are entirely justified. However, the results could be improved by treating the underlying androgen deficiency.

The *well-proportioned* mesterolone treatment acts on all the degraded structures. Therefore, a biological study is necessary for each person. The appropriate amounts vary according to each man's constitution.

Today, we are in the era of twenty-first-century medicine, computerized, scientific medicine. Biological results must be visualized in tables to understand the coordination of elements at a given time and their evolution over time.

These data are explained in detail to the person being treated. Cooperation between the doctor and patient is essential. The patient will be able to participate by reviewing the results table. The consultation lasts forty-five minutes to one hour. It occurs every 3 months until the coordinated hormonal biology is correct, according to the data. Then, the control is done every six months. If everything is correct, one visits the doctor once a year. Therapy is for life.

It takes at least ten years of practice to experience this treatment. Indeed, the stabilized patient requires only 10 specialized medical visits over 10 years. However, the experience could be faster for a physician working in a dedicated center that sees many patients. Therefore, the ability to compare data with computerized tables is significant and essential.

Male hormones are not aspirin. The androgenic disease of andropause, like any disease, requires medical treatment from the referring physician. Physicians will always seek expert advice from an endocrinologist when needed.

Analyses

Since 1974, reference laboratories have developed radioimmunoassay methods and performed hierarchical measurements with precision. If the laboratory is changed, it is preferable not to switch to a different laboratory to carry out the controls, because the methods of analysis may differ from one laboratory to another. If the laboratory changes, the biological tables must be redone to comply with the new laboratory's standards.

Medication

Mesterolone, synthesized in 1934 and introduced for medical use in 1967, is the treatment for the androgenic disease of andropause. Its formulation, marketed for over twenty-five years, is no longer protected by a patent. It is still used under many brand names today and is available in Canada, Mexico, the United Kingdom, Australia, and worldwide, except for the United States.

We should wonder why pharmaceutical companies have no interest in marketing drugs that can prevent the diseases of ageing? At the same time, the world market needs to sell cholesterol-lowering, antidiabetic, antihypertensive, antirheumatic, and antidepressant drugs. Human beings need those drugs for the moment because they have not been treated in the past to prevent diseases of ageing.

The treatment of androgenic andropause disease is done with mesterolone only. None of the testosterone's many derivatives, nor testosterone itself, has the molecular features necessary to treat male androgenetic disease. According to the Food and Drug Administration, testosterone can be used to treat **true hypogonadism**, i.e., when testosterone levels are at **castrated levels** (50 nanograms per hundred milliliters of serum). Such cases are rare. Testosterone is contraindicated in the treatment of androgenic disease, while mesterolone can treat hypogonadism, Bayer, 2007-2009 (17).

The Food and Drug Administration (FDA) Concern and "The Age-Related Hypogonadism", 2015 [18]

Testosterone products have been approved by the Food and Drug Administration (FDA) for replacement therapy in men with "classic hypogonadism" — primary or secondary hypogonadism caused by specific, well-recognized medical conditions, such as Klinefelter syndrome, pituitary injury, or toxic damage to the testicles. Those cases are rare (see page 26).

"In recent years, however, testosterone use has increased markedly among middle-aged and elderly men for a controversial condition that the FDA calls "age-related hypogonadism." This condition, also referred to as "late-onset hypogonadism," is typically diagnosed in men who, for no discernable reason other than advanced age, have serum testosterone concentrations below the normal range for healthy young men, as well as signs and symptoms that may or may not be caused by low testosterone concentrations".

"Age-related hypogonadism" and "late-onset hypogonadism" are wrong designations for a little-known or unknown disease: the "Androgenic Disease in Man", which is not a hypogonadism [16].

After the FDA, "Low T" implies treatment benefits that lack substantial evidence from controlled trials.

The FDA believes the health of American men will be well served by accurate drug labels and reliable data to inform clinical decision-making.

Until now, the mistake has been to use terms like "low testosterone" or "age-related hypogonadism, which are not diseases but imprecise concepts that have led to "therapeutic" disasters. It would have been easier to identify and treat the androgenic disease in men with mesterolone, a simple, safe, and inexpensive treatment unrecognised for fifty years [16].

Longevity, Ageing Diseases and the Pharmaceutical Industry

The Greenland shark can live up to 200 years, possibly up to 500. The giant tortoise of the Galapagos can live almost 200 years. The oldest tortoise known was named Harriet. A female brought to a zoo in Queensland, Australia, died in 2006 at the age of 176. Jeanne Calment was a French centenarian known as the longest-lived person in history when she reached 122 years and 164 days.

If Jeanne Calment lived to 122, it was because she was not affected by an ageing disease. These diseases are caused by biochemical alterations that occur after age 40, depending on the individual.

The first diseases of ageing to appear after the age of forty are the androgenic diseases of andropause and menopause. These untreated diseases limit life expectancy in the US to about 76 years for men. Today's medicine cannot ignore these diseases, as they can be identified by simple biological tests and treated with inexpensive mesterolone. The lack of prevention of ageing diseases is costing the healthcare system a fortune and is putting non-recovering patients back into circulation. At the same time, simple and inexpensive prevention through mesterolone would already make it possible to prevent certain ageing diseases, even for the poorest. This means that the prevention of ageing begins now and is the physician's business.

The pharmaceutical industry is the business of pharmacists who promise to prevent ageing within two decades, thus confusing longevity with diseases of ageing.

The billions invested in the pharmaceutical industry today and in ageing research think they are increasing longevity by ignoring the treatments of ageing diseases that already exist and are physicians' business.

Longevity can only be prolonged when ageing diseases are eliminated through prevention that already exists, is inexpensive, and available to all.

The pharmaceutical industry's search for the elixir of life or the Holy Grail of youth will take another two decades, according to the most experienced pharmacists. But medical prevention starts now. Without this prevention, pharmaceutical research will fail.

In any case, the prevention of age-related diseases will always be a matter for physicians.

Health Insurance

Health insurance services, performance, and profits will increasingly benefit from the dissemination of up-to-date medical information via the Internet. Insurers can also propose insurance programs (e.g., life insurance) based on scientific results that will modify mortality tables [13]. Health and life insurance in the 21st century will be based on medical departments that specialize in preventing age-related diseases, integrated into medical structures worldwide.

Education

The interest of the new generations of physicians in the clinical and therapeutic concepts confirmed over the years by the most severe scientific publications has been noted.

The teaching of these principles, described in this book, has not yet been integrated into traditional university training. Many years, or even generations of teachers, will still be necessary to explain to medical students the pathology of the androgenic disease of andropause, its causes and consequences in preventing ageing conditions. It is essential to teach teachers first.

The Georges Debled, MD Research Foundation, aims to disseminate the teaching of the clinical and therapeutic principles of Dr Georges Debled, not only to the medical profession but also to men who want to understand their ageing problems.

The Foundation's website is constantly updated. It allows everyone to understand the elements of health problems related to diseases of ageing, especially their initial causes. I have published the principles set out in this book in the medical press, in the general media, at numerous congresses, and on television and radio networks since 1974. The Foundation's website lists these works. It is the expression of a conceptual series in continuous development.

Clinical and scientific research is an essential element of anti-ageing treatments.

In clinical practice, the replacement of diseased cells with stem cells, genetic corrections, and the substitution of anti-ageing "factors" must always consider the pathology and treatment of androgenic andropause disease since longevity is significantly reduced when androgens are lacking [13]. The studies to be carried out will be considerable.

The Spanish Society of Anti-Ageing and Longevity Medicine (SEMAL) has been continuously disseminating advances in the fight against ageing diseases for 20 years, thanks to its President, Dr José Márquez Serres. And thanks to the efforts of Manuel del Castillo, Professor of Medical Physiology at the Faculty of Medicine of the University of Granada, and President of the SEMAL Scientific Committee. Professor Antonio Ayala of the Department of Biochemistry and Molecular Biology at the University of Seville, and Vice-President of the Society, provides scientific assistance to the SEMAL, which is probably the most advanced medical society today in teaching anti-ageing medicine.

A Tsunami of Ageing Diseases

We may be witnessing a tsunami of diseases of ageing. Among these diseases, dementia occupies a worrying place. As the world's population ages, the World Health Organization (WHO) predicts that the number of people with dementia will triple from 50 million today to 82 million in 2030 and 152 million in 2050.

Given that the diseases of ageing develop over forty years and lead to death, it can be predicted that by 2060, we will see the extinction of a specific population of women and men who will not have received preventive treatment for the diseases of ageing.

The annual cost of dementia worldwide is approximately $818 billion. By 2030, this cost will more than double to US$2 trillion. There are currently ten million new cases of dementia each year, as the prevention of this disease of ageing is not yet standard practice.

Anti-ageing therapy includes the treatment of androgenic diseases of menopause and andropause [4-7; 14-16; 19-27]. This treatment can prevent, among other things, the development of arteriosclerosis, which is responsible for most dementia cases.

Treatment of androgenic diseases of menopause and andropause is available and inexpensive. The results are most effective with a balanced diet.

All diseases described in this book depend wholly or partly on mesterolone supplementation. This therapy, told here for the first time, prevents arteriosclerosis, an aggravating cause of Parkinson's and Alzheimer's.

As we age, all our structures shrink. But mesterolone prevents connective tissue sclerosis, which reduces all movement.

Preventing arterial sclerosis will also prevent one from ending one's life blind or deaf.

When the tsunami of ageing diseases arrives, it will be too late.

The method to calculate the exact amount of mesterolone you need is now described in Prostate Ageing Control [27].

Prevention of ageing diseases is relevant to the medicine of the twenty-first century. The Georges Debled Research Foundation is dedicated to research on ageing diseases.

www.georgesdebled.org

Thank you for your interest.

Conclusion:
Ageless Man

With the knowledge of hormones, are we not the day before to get the hand on the development of our body—and of the brain itself?

—*Teilhard de Chardin,*
The Human Phenomenon

Grow Young Again:

How to Cure and Prevent Diseases of Ageing

Since the end of the seventeenth century, life for humans has not changed much. But yes, one notes a progressive lengthening of longevity, and one speaks of a fourth, and even a fifth and sixth, age. This remarkable phenomenon results from the fulgurating progress of medicine over the past fifty years, when one lived, on average, twenty years less than today.

The androgenic disease of andropause and senility provokes devastation that puts healthcare systems in danger.

The untreated androgenic disease of andropause causes a progressive reduction in sexual capacities and starts the vicious cycle of self-destruction, leading to death. Considerable sums are necessary today to fight against the diseases of ageing. But medical technology seems condemned to save fewer patients by neglecting the prevention of their organs' degeneration.

The traditional conception of cardiovascular disease is unaware of the essential principle of vital energy sources. The years that precede cardiac arrest or fatal arterial thrombosis are lived with multiple and dramatic incidents. The economic and social costs of cardiovascular disease are gigantic, comprising the most significant financial burden of the healthcare economy. Degenerative cardiovascular diseases are never cured. They are looked after and operated on, but patients have relapses and worsen unrelentingly.

The cardiac patient increasingly depends on medical technology. Cardiac transplants are spectacular but do not last. The new heart, grafted into a man with an androgenic disease of andropause, degenerates with the receiver's body, with the coronary arteries obstructing it quickly. How is it that traditional therapy for cardiovascular disease does not consider the energy sources necessary for the contractions of the musculature, heart, and arteries? Glycogen and contractile proteins constitute the energy needed for the arterial and cardiac muscle to function, thanks to male hormones. Degeneration of the heart and blood vessels results from a lack of energy. The heart's contraction weakens in their absence, the arteries narrow, and the veins become varicose. Even if an artificial heart replaces the diseased heart, the whole of the body degenerates.

A lack of energetic factors affects blood composition: the number of red blood cells falls, cholesterol and blood sugar levels rise, and blood fluidity (antithrombin III) decreases. For example, a man with an androgenic disease of andropause has a weak heart that propels his fatty and viscous blood through narrowed arteries. He takes all kinds of drugs to regulate his heart, reduce his hypertension, thin his blood, and lower his sugar and cholesterol levels. All those functions can be carried out naturally by male hormones.

The excess weight of the population continues to increase overall and regularly, causing an increasingly high death rate due to ignorance of food guidelines. Certain men, conscious of their excess weight, make desperate efforts to find a classic silhouette, increasingly necessary in a society that eliminates those who do not impress. Many slimming regimes are difficult to follow because they do not account for the role of male hormones in regulating fat and sugar metabolism. In a state of perpetual imbalance, some individuals abandon diets altogether. Thus, they end up resembling a fat grandfather, without hope of living longer than he did.

Eye and hearing troubles, widespread after age fifty, are closely related to the degeneration of sense organs; one can no longer be unaware of the role of male hormones in their integrity and structure.

By 1974, I described the mechanism of sexual ageing (chapters 6–9). Preventive medication with mesterolone makes it possible to preserve a healthy erection and ejaculation.

Prostate diseases are the direct consequence of androgenic disease of andropause. Prostate surgery can be done on an open belly. Finer, and consequently less traumatic, surgery is performed by endoscopy when there are urinary difficulties. The prostatism of androgenic disease of andropause is caused by the disordered state of sex hormone balance. One can, today, stabilize prostate hypertrophy by balancing sex hormones, thus delaying or avoiding the moment of surgery.

Osteoarthritis is an infirmity of senescence. It is invalidating and painful, and its medical and social costs burden healthcare budgets. Orthopedic surgery repairs the joint articulations of older and disabled men. Prostheses can replace practically all joints. Individuals are even assisted today by successive, perilous hip prostheses replacements. Unfortunately, the damage is severe, and patients are often uneasy about reparative surgery.

Care for arthritis requires an entire industry. It deploys battalions of doctors and medical staff, though it is true that treating symptoms never cures osteoarthritis.

Osteoporosis and degenerative changes are closely associated with a lack of male hormones. In their absence, patients will experience new articular blockings and other fractures in a process that will not end.

Lastly, depression and melancholy in men with an androgenic disease of andropause are frequent and lead to their retirement around age sixty. Their brains, deprived of male hormones, cannot meet the demands of the external world. Ousted from social and economic structures, they have no future, whereas their human and professional resources could be useful if they were to recover their vital energy.

Metamorphosis and Rebirth of Men beyond Age Forty

Formerly, due to ignorance and fatalism, the aged accepted the diseases of ageing—one aged without hope of better days. Reduction in sexual activity inevitably led to a lack of libido. One did not speak about it. Death was premature. Things were just so.

Many men still think they cannot change any aspect of their ageing, mainly because of a lack of information.

Since the end of the Second World War, scientific knowledge has made extraordinary progress. Computers exceed the capacities of the human brain. Researchers work on genes in the hope of eliminating genetic diseases. In short, all seems possible.

During this time, however, men degenerate in the millions, endangering the balance of societies. This phenomenon is paradoxical and, according to current knowledge, completely anachronistic. Certain men are conscious of that. Suffering from troubles of andropause, whereas all was well a few months before, they cannot accept the idea that medical science cannot cure them; they have questioned this a hundred times. Therefore, while wanting to live in good health, they do not ask for anything more than a life supplement.

It is necessary to reactivate their biological program, which has reached its average duration.

Replacement of the missing male hormones restarts sexual activity and prolongs the biological mechanisms of life. Therefore, good sexual activity and the absence of andropause troubles reflect good health.

The general degradations appear around age forty, with a moderate rise in blood pressure, some excess weight, a craving for sugar, an increase in blood cholesterol, minor cardiac symptoms, and stiffness of movement.

Very often, the silhouette has already changed and is a sign that does not mislead.

Male hormones act on the various structures of the organism. Sharp observers understand that health concerns the whole of the body. Is there hope? Undoubtedly. The metamorphosis is possible. Men with an androgenic disease of andropause can change, just as the caterpillar becomes the chrysalis.

The second surprise is that he must increase his consciousness and acquire more soul for that to occur. To take hormones to live longer without better living is entirely contradictory. Vital efforts are necessary to understand and implement rigorous control of food, harmonious physical exercise, oxygenation, and relaxation. This program, however simple, often runs counter to monolithic habits. After reflection, change happens little by little.

The third surprise is the complete metamorphosis at the end of the road. In full possession of mental faculties, the regenerated man can finally release himself from material contingencies, a requirement of true rebirth. The chrysalis becomes a butterfly.

Ageless Man

The treatment and prevention of diseases of ageing will have a considerable impact on the social, economic, and cultural spheres, as the human life cycle will change.

Today, the regressive man can only truly realise himself between twenty and forty years. He then regresses unrelentingly up to eighty years. The times of the backward man are now the times of the ageless man.

With knowledge and hormones, today's men can prevent sexual ageing, which precedes senile involution and many diseases. As a result, they will no longer suffer from the androgenic disease of andropause, senescence, and decline. "Just be" will be his reason to live.

The ageless man lives a continued revitalization. But unfortunately, one cannot estimate his longevity.

We are still unaware of where the long-term treatment of sexual ageing and other biological ageing will lead. We will eventually combine cell regeneration treatments with the knowledge of nucleic acids and cell "mothers" that condition cellular division.

Genetic research has made significant progress. Soon, it will complement the dynamic biochemistry of the androgenic disease of andropause *and menopause.*

A formidable race begins to control one's lifetime from this time on. The future of men is closely related to knowledge of the biological mechanisms of the male body, as described in this book. Therefore, the digitalization of all physiological parameters of each person must be standard.

To reach the stage of ageless man, we will also have to beat cancer. In 2025, an estimated 2,041,910 new cases of cancer will be diagnosed in the United States, and 618,120 people will die from the disease. Considerable progress has already been made in understanding the control points in cancer cells that can be targeted to block cell proliferation.

However, if all cancers were cured, the body's deterioration in the absence of prevention of androgenic disease in men from age 40 onwards would prolong the lives of organisms severely weakened by arteriosclerosis, cardiovascular disease, osteoarthritis, and Alzheimer's disease.

The prevention of diseases of ageing is already possible. Revitalization with mesterolone after age 40 is necessary to prevent decline. Other biological deficiencies that should appear later will be considered. Prevention is the principal future activity for new medical professionals. Correcting Alzheimer's disease at seventy years of age is almost impossible. It is at age forty that research and prevention must begin.

Regressive Man	**Ageless Man**
Birth	Birth
Childhood	Childhood
Adolescence	Adolescence
Adulthood	
Androgenic Disease of Andropause	Adulthood
Senescence	
Senility	
Death	?

The Ageless Man is already born. Do you want to be him? Think and act now.

Updated January 12, 2026

Bibliography

1

Sexual Ageing Announces the Degeneration of all Structures of the Organism

1. SEYMOUR Fl., DUFFY C., KOERNER A., "A Case of Authenticated Fertility in Man of 94", JAMA, 105, 1935, p. 1423-1425

2. DEBLED G.- L'Andropause, cause, conséquences et remèdes. Maloine, Paris, 1988.

3. DEBLED G. The androgenic disease of andropause. SEMAL congress, Seville, October 5, 2019.

4. MORER-FARGAS F. und NOWAKOWSKI H. -Die Testosteronausscheidung im Harn bei Männlichen Individuen: Acta Endocrinologica, 49: 443-452, 1965

2

Male Hormones, the Keys to Andropause

1. ROBEL P. -Mode d'Action des Androgènes : Les Androgènes. Rapports présentés à la XVe réunion des endocrinologistes de langue française : 20-38. Athènes, 6-8 septembre 1979. -MASSON PARIS NEW YORK BARCELONE MILAN 1979.

2. MICHEL G., BAULIEU E.E., et COURRIER R. -Récepteur Cytosoluble des Androgènes dans un Muscle Strié Squelettique : C.R. Acad. Sc. Paris, 279: 421-424, 1974.

3. BLASIUS R., KAFER K., SEITZ W. - Untersuchungen über die Wirkung von Testosteron auf die Kontraktilen Strukturproteine des Herzens. Klin. Woch., 34, 11/12, 324, 1956.

4. AL MADHOUN AS, VORONOVA A, RYAN T, ZAKARIYAH A, MCINTIRE C, GIBSON L, SHELTON M, RUEL M, SKERJANC IS. Testosterone enhances cardiomyogenesis in stem cells and recruits the Androgen Receptor to the MEF2C and HCN4 genes. J Mol Cell Cardiol. 2013 Apr 15. Elsevier Ltd.

5. RODRIGO T. CALADO, WILLIAM T. YEWDELL, KEISHA L. WILKERSON, JOSHUA A. REGAL, SACHIKO KAJIGAYA, CONSTANTINE A. STRATAKIS, AND NEAL S. YOUNG. Sex hormones, acting on the TERT gene, increase telomerase activity in human primary hematopoietic cells. Blood. 2009 Sep 10; 114 (11): 2236-2243

6. PURIFOY F.E., KOOPMANS L.H., MAYES D.M. -Age Differences in Serum Androgen Levels in Normal Adult Males: Human Biol., 53: 499-511, 1981.

7. GRAY A, BERLIN JA, MCKINLAY JB, et al. An examination of research design effects on the association of testosterone and male ageing: results of a meta-analysis. J Clin Epidemiol 1991; 44: 671-84.

8. REBECCA L FERRINLL AND ELIZABETH BARRETT-CONNOR. Sex Hormones and Age: A Cross-sectional Study of Testosterone and Estradiol and Their Bioavailable Fractions in Community-dwelling Men.
Am. Journal of Epidemiology, 1998; 147:750-4.

9. HENRY A. FELDMAN, CHRISTOPHER LONGCOPE, CAROL A. DERBY, CATHERINE B. JOHANNES, ANDRE B. ARAUJO, ANDREA D. COVIELLO, WILLIAM J. BREMNER, AND JOHN B. Mc KINLAY. Age Trends in the Level of Serum Testosterone and Other Hormones in Middle-Aged Men: Longitudinal Results from the Massachusetts Male Ageing Study. Journal of Clinical Endocrinology & Metabolism, 2002; 87(2): 589—98.

3
The Castrato, A Model of Androgenic disease of andropause

1. PITTARD E. – La castration chez l'homme et les modifications morphologiques qu'elle entraîne- Recherches sur les adeptes d'une secte mystique, les Skoptzy, MASSON PARIS 1934.

4
Treatment with Male Hormones is an Old Concept

1. BROWN-SEQUARD, F.R.S. & c., Note on the effects produced on man by subcutaneous injections of a liquid obtained from the testicles of animals: The Lancet, 105-107, 29 July 1889

2. VORONOFF S. -La Greffe Testiculaire de Singe à l'Homme. GASTON DOIN et Cie. PARIS 1930.

3. MILLER N.E., HUBERT, GILBERT, and HAMILTON J.B. -Mental and Behavior Changes Following Male Hormone Treatment of Adult Castration, Hypogonadism, and Psychic Impotence: Proc. Soc. Exper. Biol. & Med., 38: 538- 540, 1938.

4. WERNER A.A. The Male Climacteric: J.A.M.A., 15 April: 1441-1443, 1939.

5. HELLER C.G., MEYERS G.B., The Male Climacteric, its Symptomatology, Diagnosis, and treatment: J.A.MA., 126: 472-477, 1944.

6. BRUCHOVSKY N. and WILSON J.D., The Conversion of Testosterone to 5α-Androstan-17β-ol-3-one by Rat Prostate in Vivo and in Vitro. The Journal of Biological Chemistry. Vol. 243, Nº 8, Issue of April 25, pp2012-2021, 1968

7. ANDERSON K.M. and SHUTSUNG LIAO, Selective Retention of Dihydrotestosterone by Prostatic Nuclei. Nature 219, 277-279 (20 July 1968) ; doi :10. 1038/219277a0

8. DEBLED G.- L'Andropause, cause, conséquences et remèdes. Maloine, Paris, 1988.

9. DEBLED G. Andropause. 1 : Le castrat : un modèle "expérimental". N° 4308 - 24 mai 1989. Le Quotidien du Médecin. Paris.

10. DEBLED G. Andropause 2 : Dépister pour reculer le vieillissement prématuré. N° 43 l 3 - 3 l mai 1989. Le Quotidien du Médecin. Paris.

11. DEBLED G. Andropause 3 : Sclérose des corps caverneux : le fatalisme n'est plus de mise. N° 4318 - 7 juin 1989. Le Quotidien du Médecin. Paris.

12. DEBLED G. Andropause 4 : Les troubles "émotionnels" ne doivent pas cacher l'impuissance organique. N° 4323 - 14 juin 1989. Le Quotidien du Médecin. Paris.

13. DEBLED G. Andropause 5 : Les troubles de l'éjaculation. N° 4328 - 21 juin 1989. Le Quotidien du Médecin. Paris.

14. DEBLED G. Andropause 6 : Les perturbations de la miction. N° 4334 - 29 juin 1989. Le Quotidien du Médecin. Paris.

15. DEBLED G. Andropause 7 : L'atrophie de la prostate. N° 4372 - 26 septembre 1989. Le Quotidien du Médecin. Paris. Le Quotidien du Médecin. Paris.

16. DEBLED G. Andropause 8 : Des difficultés mictionnelles à l'insuffisance rénale. N° 4377 - 3 octobre 1989. Le Quotidien du Médecin. Paris.

17. DEBLED G. Andropause 9 : Un âge où "tout se dégrade". N° 4382 - 10 octobre 1989. Le Quotidien du Médecin. Paris.

18. DEBLED G. Andropause 10 : Les hormones sexuelles de l'homme. N4337 - 17 octobre l 989. Le Quotidien du Médecin. Paris.

19. DEBLED G. Andropause 11 : Le généraliste et l'exploration du vieillissement sexuel. N° 4397 - 31 octobre 1989. Le Quotidien du Médecin. Paris.

20. DEBLED G. Andropause 12 : Les androgènes favorisent-ils l'apparition d'un cancer de la prostate ? N° 4401 - 7 novembre 1989. Le Quotidien du Médecin. Paris.

21. DEBLED G. Andropause 13 : Le traitement hormonal. N° 4422 - 6 décembre 1989. Le Quotidien du Médecin. Paris.

22. DEBLED G. Au-delà de celle limite votre ticket est toujours valables. Albin Michel. 1992.Paris.

23. DEBLED G. The male climacteric prime cause of sex involution. The Tenth annual international symposium on man and his environment in health and disease. February 27-March 1, 1992. Dallas. Texas. The U.S.A.

24. DEBLED G. The male climacteric prime cause of ageing. The Tenth annual international symposium on man and his environment in health and disease. February 27-March 1, 1992. Dallas. Texas. The U.S.A.

25. DEBLED G. Le traitement hormonal du vieillissement sexuel de l'homme. Journal de médecine esthétique et de chirurgie dermatologique. Vol XXII- N° 85: 7 - 16, 1995

26. DEBLED G. La enfermedad "andropausia". Congreso internacional de medicina antienvejecimiento. Septiembre 21-22 y 23 de 2006 Club Militar de Bogotá. Bogotá D.C.

27. DEBLED G. Atrofia de la próstata y envejecimiento. Congreso internacional de medicina antienvejecimiento. Septiembre 21-22 y 23 de 2006 Club Militar de Bogotá. Bogotá D.C.

28. DEBLED G. La enfermedad "andropausia". Mi experiencia hace 32 años. International congress of anti-ageing Medicine Vº congreso de la sociedad española de medicina antienvejecimiento y longevidad. Madrid 3,4 y 5 de noviembre 2006. Hotel Melia Castilla. Madrid.

29. DOMINIQUE SIMON, MARIE-ALINE CHARLES, KHALIL NAHOUL, GENEVIEVE ORSSAUD, JACQUELINE KREJNSKI, VERONIQUE HULLY, EVELYNE JOUBERT, LAURE PAPOZ AND EVELINE ESCHWEGE. Association between Plasma Total Testosterone and Cardiovascular Risk Factors in Healthy Adult Men: The Telecom Study. Clin. Endocrinol. Metab.1997 82: 682-685, doi: 10.1210/jc.82.2.682

30. BANSAL V.P., Professor, and Head, Department of Orthopedics, Universal College of Medical Sciences & Teaching Hospital, Bhairahawa, Nepal. MS Orth (Punjab). M Ch Orth (Liverpool). DPMR (Mumbai). Andropause a clinical entity. Journal of Universal College of Medical Sciences (2013) Vol 1 Nº 02, 54-68.

5
A Vigorous Longevity Beyond Eighty Years

1. NIESCHLAG E. -The Endocrine Function of the Human Testes regarding Sexuality.: Sex. Hormon. Behav., 62: 183-207, 1979.

6
Premature Sexual Ageing

1. LI F, YUE H, YAMAGUCHI K, OKADA K, MATSUSHITA K, ANDO M, CHIBA K, FUJISAWA M. Effect of surgical repair on testosterone production in infertile men with varicocele: a meta-analysis. Int. J Urol. 2012 Feb; 19(2):149-54.

7
"Emotional" Disorders should not hide Organic Impotence

1. PEARLMAN C.K. and KOBASHI L.I. -Frequency of Intercourse in Men: J. Urol., 107: 298-301, 1972.

8
Ejaculation Disorders

1. PEARLMAN C.K. and KOBASHI L.I. -Frequency of Intercourse in Men: J. Urol., 107: 298-301, 1972.

9
Prostate Problems

1. ROUVIERE H. et DELMAS A. -Anatomie Humaine. Tome 2: 592. 12ème Edition Révisée et Augmentée   MASSON PARIS NEW-YORK BARCELONE MILAN MEXICO SAO PAULO 1985.

2. CHEVREMONT M. -Cytologie et Histologie : p.865-867 Editions DESOER, LIEGE 1956.

3. DEBLED G. L'Hyperoestrogénie Associée à la Dysectasie Fibreuse de l'Urètre Prostatique : Bulletins et Mémoires de la Société de Médecine de Paris, 7 : 199-204, 1980.

4. DEBLED G. -La Pathologie obstructive Congénitale de l'Uretère Terminal - Thèse d'agrégation de l'enseignement supérieur en Sciences Urologiques, Université Libre de Bruxelles, 18 Mai 1971 : Acta Urol. Belg., 39: 371-465, 1971.

5. GREGOIR W. et DEBLED G. -Méga-Uretère Congénital : Encyclopédie Médico-Chirurgicale, 18, Rue SEGUIER. PARIS VIe 18158 E10: 4-14 1971.

6. FDA Drug Safety Communication: 5-alpha reductase inhibitors (5-AR1s) may increase the risk of a more serious form of prostate cancer. 6-9-2011.

7. MEEKER AK, SOMMERFELD HJ, COFFEY DS. Telomerase is activated in the prostate and seminal vesicles of the castrated rat. Endocrinology 1996 Dec. 137(12):5743-6.

8. EDWARDS C.N., STEINTHORSSON E. and NICHOLSON D. -An Autopsy Study of Latent Prostatic Carcinoma: Cancer, 6: 531, 1953.

9. FRANKS L.M. -Latent Carcinoma of the Prostate: J. Path. Bact., 68: 603, 1954.

10. Mc. NEAL J.E., BOSTWICK D.G., KINRACHUK R.A., REDWINE E.A., FREIHA F.S., and STAMEY T.A. -Patterns on Progression in Prostate Cancer: Lancet, 1: 60, 1986.

11. ZARIDGE G. and BOYLE P. -Cancer of the Prostate: Epidemiology and Etiology: Br. J. Urol., 59, 4: 493-502, 1987

12. NORUMA A., HEILBRUN L.K., STEMMERMANN G.N., and JUDD H.L. - Prediagnostic Serum Hormones and the Risk of Prostate Cancer: Cancer Research, 48: 3515-3517, 1988.

13. Mc MAHON M.J., BUTLER A.V.J., and THOMAS G.H. -Morphological Responses of Prostatic Carcinoma to Testosterone in Organ Culture: Br. J. Cancer, 26: 388-394, 1972.

14. VETERANS ADMINISTRATION COOPERATIVE UROLOGICAL RESEARCH GROUP (VACURG) -Treatment and Survival of Patients with Cancer of the Prostate: Surg. Gynecol. Obstet., 124: 1011-1017, 1967.

15. LABRIE F., DUPONT A. et BELANGER A. -Un Nouveau Traitement du Cancer de la Prostate : La Suppression Complète des Androgènes- In MAUVAIS-JARVIS P., SCHAISON G., BOUCHARD P., MAHOUDEAU J. et LABRIE F. -Médecine de la Reproduction Masculine : 367-383 FLAMMARION MEDECINE SCIENCES PARIS 1984.

16. PROUT G.R. Jr. and BREWER W.R. -Response of Men with Advanced Prostatic Carcinoma to Exogenous Administration of Testosterone: Cancer, 20: 1871-1877, 1967.

17. MORALES A., CONNOLLY J.G., and BRUCE A.W. -Androgen Therapy in Advanced Carcinoma of the Prostate: Can. Med. Assoc. J., 105; 1: 71-72, 1971.

18. DEBLED G. Los efectos adversos de los inhibidores de la 5-alfa-reductasa. SEMAL: 2nd International congress anti-ageing medicine. Miami, February 6th to 9th 2020.

19. DEBLED G. Composition for the treatment of cancers. OPRI (Office belge de la propriété intellectuelle) : 100075876. Nº 2020/5139. March 02 2020.

10
Diabetes and Androgenic disease of andropause

1. DANAEI G, FINUCANE MM, LU Y, SINGH GM, COWAN MJ, PACIOREK CJ ET AL. National, regional, and global trends in fasting plasma glucose and diabetes prevalence since 1980: systematic analysis of health examination surveys and epidemiological studies with 370 country years and 2.7 million participants. Lancet, 2011, 378(9785):31–40.

2. WORLD HEALTH ORGANIZATION. Global health risks. Mortality and burden of disease are attributable to selected major risks. Geneva, 2009.

3. PELLEGRINI G. -L'Azione Antidiabetica degli Ormoni Sessuali Maschili nel quadro della Fisiopatologia del Diabete: Minerva Medica, 27: 1-9, 1947.

4. ANDO S., RUBENS R., and ROTTIERS R. -Androgen Plasma Levels in Male Diabetics: J. Endocrinol. Invest., 7: 21-24, 1984.

5. MOELLER J. -Cholesterol: 27 SPRINGER-VERLAG BERLIN HEIDELBERG NEW YORK LONDON PARIS TOKYO 1987.

6. DOMINIQUE SIMON, MD, PHD, MARIE-ALINE CHARLES, MD, NAJIBA LAHLOU, MD, KHALIL NAHOUL, MD, JEAN-MICHEL OPPERT, MD, PHD, MICHE` LE GOUAULT-HEILMANN, MD, NICOLE LEMORT, BSC, NADINE

THIBULT, BSC, EVELYNE JOUBERT, MD, BEVERLEY BALKAU, PHD, EVELINE ESCHWEGE, MD: Androgen Therapy Improves Insulin Sensitivity and Decreases Leptin Level in Healthy Adult Men with Low Plasma Total Testosterone. DIABETES CARE, VOLUME 24, NUMBER 12, DECEMBER 2001

7. JIN YOUNG SHIN, EUN KI PARK1, BYOUNG JIN PARK, JAE YONG SHIM, HYE REE LEE. High-normal Glucose Levels in Non-diabetic and Pre-Diabetic Men Are Associated with Decreased Testosterone Levels. Korean J Fam Med. 2012; 33:152-156.

11

Male Hormones Against Cholesterol

1. LIPID RESEARCH PROGRAM -The Lipid Research Clinics Population Studies Data Book -NIH Publication No 80: 1527, vol 1 BETHESDA, 1980.

2. DAI W.S., MD, DrPH, GUTAI J.P., MD, KULLER L.H., MD, DrPH, LAPORTE R.E., PhD., FALVO-GERARD L., MPH, and GAGGIULA A., Ph.D. - Relation between Plasma High-Density Lipoprotein Cholesterol and Sex Hormone Concentrations in Men: Am. J. Cardiol., 53: 1259-1263, 1984.

3. GUTAI J., LAPORTE R., KULLER J., DAI W., FALVO-GERARD L., CAGGIULA A. Plasma Testosterone, High-Density Lipoprotein Cholesterol, and other Lipoprotein Fractions: Am. J. Cardiol., 48: 897-902, 1981.

4. CHADDA J.S., TERAN A-Z., FELDMAN E.B., and GREENBLATT R.B.: Lipoprotein Studies in Climacteric Men Treated with Pure Testosterone: Maturitas, 6, 2: 97, 1984.

5. BREIER Ch., DREXEL H., LISCH H.-J., MÜHLBERGER V., HEROLD M., and KNAPP E. -Essential Role of Post-Heparin Lipoprotein Lipase Activity and of Plasma Testosterone in Coronary Artery Disease: The Lancet, June 1: 1242-1244, 1985.

6. HOFMAN A, OTT A, BRETELER MM, BOTS ML, SLOOTER AJ, VAN HARSKAMP F, VAN DUIJN CN, VAN BROECKHOVEN C, GROBBEE DE.- Atherosclerosis, apolipoprotein E, and prevalence of dementia and Alzheimer's disease in the Rotterdam Study. Lancet. 1997 Jan 18;349(9046):151-4.

12

Excess Weight and Obesity: The Ideal Weight

1. LEW E.A. and GARFINKEL L. -Variations in Mortality by Weight among 750.000 Men and Women -J. Chron. Dis., 32: 563, 1979.

2. ZUMOFF B., STRAIN G.W., MILLER L.K., ROSNER W., SENIE R., SERES D.S., and ROSENFELD R.S. -Plasma Free and Non-Sex-Binding-Globulin-Bound Testosterone Are Decreased in Obese Men in Proportion to their Degree of Obesity: J. Clin. Endocrinol. Metabol., 71,4: 929-931, 1990

3. HEUFELDER AE, SAAD F, BUNCK MC, GOOREN L. Fifty-two-week treatment with diet and exercise plus transdermal testosterone reverses the metabolic syndrome and improves glycemic control in men with newly diagnosed type 2 diabetes and subnormal plasma testosterone. J Androl 2009; 30: 726-33

4. FARID SAAD, ANTONIO AVERSA, ANDREA M. ISIDORI, LOUIS J. GOOREN. Testosterone as Potential Effective Therapy in Treatment of Obesity in Men with Testosterone Deficiency: A Review. Current Diabetes Reviews, 2012, 8, 131-143.13

13

Muscular Weakness

1. FORSTER D.W. - Diabète Sucré, 327 : 1778 dans HARRISON T.R.- Principes de Médecine Interne MEDECINE-SCIENCES FLAMMARION PARIS 1989.

2. BOREL J-P., RANDOUX A., MAQUARTF-X., LE PEUCH C., VALEYRE J.- Biochimie Dynamique -1421 : 1400. MALOINE DECARIE PARIS MONTREAL 1987.

3. JUNG I. and BEAULIEU E-E. -Testosterone Cytosol Receptor in the Rat Levator Ani Muscle: Nature New Biology, 237: 24-26, 1972.

4. GILLESPIE C.A. and EDGERTON V.R. -The role of Testosterone in Exercise-induced Glycogen Supercompensation: Horm. Metab. Res., 2: 364-366, 1970.

5. PLAS F. -Variations de la Fonction Androgénique au cours des Efforts Prolongés : Bull. Acad. Nat. Méd., 162,6 : 494-499, 1978.

6. MORVILLE R., PESQUIES P., MAROTTE H., SERRURIER B.D. et COBRON C. - Effets d'un Apport Exogène de Dihydrotestostérone sur les Variations des Androgènes Plasmatiques au cours d'Efforts Prolongés : Médecine du Sport, 53, 2: 37-44, 1979.

7. DE LIGNIERES B. et MICHEL G. -Androgènes et Médecine Sportive- Rapport présenté à la XVème Réunion des Endocrinologistes de Langue Française. Athènes, 6-8 septembre 1979   LES ANDROGÈNES MASSON PARIS NEW YORK BARCELONE MILAN 1979.

8. SERRA C, TANGHERLINI F, RUDY S, LEE D, TORALDO G, SANDOR NL, ZHANG A, JASUJA R, BHASIN S. Testosterone improves the regeneration of old and young mouse skeletal muscle. J Gerontol A Biol Sci Med Sci. 2013 Jan; 68(1):17-26.

14

Arteriosclerosis or Arterial Rigidity

1. National Centre for Health Statistics -Vital Statistics Report, Final Mortality Statistics, 1982.

2. BEST and TAYLOR - -Physiological Basis of Medical Practice: 155 WILLIAMS and WILKINS COMPANY BALTIMORE 1950.

3. DEBLED G. -La Pathologie obstructive Congénitale de l'Uretère Terminal - Thèse d'agrégation de l'enseignement supérieur en Sciences Urologiques, Université Libre de Bruxelles, 18 mai 1971 : Acta Urol. Belg., 39 : 371-465, 1971.

4. GREGOIR W. et DEBLED G. -Méga-Uretère Congénital : Encyclopédie Médico-Chirurgicale, 18, Rue SEGUIER. PARIS VI 18158 E10 : 4-14, 1971.

5. DEBLED G. L'anatomie pathologique de l'uretère dilaté. Procès-verbaux, mémoires et discussions de l'Association Française d'Urologie, 67ème Session : 521-525, 1974

6. DEBLED G. Steroid hormone for the prevention of diseases associated with ageing. (OPRI) Office belge de la propriété intellectuelle: 100072468. Nº 2019/5905. Decembre 13, 2019.

15

Anemia

1. STEINGLASS P., GORDON A.S., CHARIPPER H.A. -Effect of Castration and Sex Hormones on Blood of the Rat: Proc. Soc. exp. Biol. Med., 48: 169-177, 1941.

2. KENNEDY B.J. and GILBERTSEN A.S. - Increased Erythropoiesis Induced by Androgenic Hormones: J. Clin. Invest. 35: 717, 1956.

3. KENNEDY B.J. - Fluoxymesterone in Advanced Breast Cancer: New Engl. J. Med., 259: 673, 1958.

4. SHAHIDI N.T. - Androgens and Erythropoiesis: N. Engl. J. Med., 289: 72-80, 1973.

5. NAJEAN Y. and coll. -Long Term Follow-up in Patients with Aplastic Anemia. A study of 137 Androgen-Treated Patients surviving more than Two Years: Am. J. Med., 71: 543-551, 1981.

6. CLAUSTRES M., BELLET H., SULTAN C.-Action des Androgènes sur les Cellules-Souches Erythroïdes en Culture : Ann. Biol. clin., 44: 5-13, 1986.

7. Luigi Ferrucci, MD, Ph.D., Marcello Maggio, MD, Stefania Bandinelli, MD, Shehzad Basaria, MD, Fulvio Lauretani, MD, Alessandro Ble, MD, Giorgio Valenti, MD, William B. Ershler, MD, Jack M. Guralnik, MD, Ph.D., and Dan L. Longo, MD. Low Testosterone Levels and the Risk of Anemia in Older Men and Women. Arch Intern Med. 2006 July 10; 166(13): 1380–1388.

16

Viscous Blood - Thromboses – Embolisms -Varicose Veins - Hemorrhoids

1. BONITHON-KOPP C., SCARABIN P.-Y., BARA L., CASTANIER M., JACQUESON A., and ROGER M. -Relationship between Sex Hormones and Haemostatic Factors in Healthy Middle-Aged Men: Artheriosclerosis, 71: 71-76, 1988.

2. CARON Ph., SIE P., BENNET A., CAMARE R., BONEU B. et LOUVET J.P. - Testosterone Plasmatique et Inhibiteur Anti Activateur Tissulaire du

Plasminogène Chez l'Homme: Ann. Endocrinol., 49, 6: 117C (182), 1988- 8ème Congrès Français d'Endocrinologie, Bruxelles 3-5 Octobre 1988.

3. FEARNLEY G.R. and CHAKRABARTI R. -Increase of Blood Fibrinolytic Activity by Testosterone: The Lancet, July 21: 128-132, 1962.

4. WALKER I.D. and DAVIDSON J.F. -Long-Trem Fibrinolytic Enhancement with Anabolic Steroid Therapy: A Five Year Study: Progress in Chemical Fibrinolysis and Thrombosis, Vol 3: 491-499. Edited by J.F. DAVIDSON, R.M. ROWAN, M.M. SAMAMA, and P.C. DESNOYERS- RAVEN PRESS NEW YORK 1978.

5. WORLD HEALTH ORGANIZATION -Prevention of Ischaemic Heart Disease. Metabolic Aspects: WHO Symposium, WHO/CVD/73:3, MADRID1972.

6. SVETLANA KALINCHENKO, ALEXANDR ZEMLYANOY, AND LOUIS GOOREN. Improvement of the diabetic foot upon testosterone administration to hypogonadal men with peripheral arterial disease. Report of three cases.

Cardiovascular Diabetology, 8: 19, 2009.

7. WIMAN B., LJUNGBERG B., CHMELIEWSKA J., URDEN G., BLOMBACK M., and JOHNSON H. -The Role of the Fibrinolytic System in Deep Vein Thrombosis: J. Lab. Clin. Med., 105: 265-270, 1985.

8. BROWSE N.L. and BURNAND K.G. -The Cause of Venous Ulceration: Lancet, II: 243-245, 1982.

9. BENNET A., CARON Ph., SIE P., LOUVET J.-P., et BAZEX J. -Ulcères de Jambe Post-Phlébitiques et Caryotype XYY: Tests de Fibrinolyse et Fonction Androgénique: Ann. Dermatol. Venereol., 114: 1097-1101, 1987.

17

Hypertension, Disease of the World

1. MERAI R, SIEGEL C, RAKOTZ M, BASCH P, WRIGHT J, WONG B; DHSC, THORPE P. CDC Grand Rounds: A Public Health Approach to Detect and Control Hypertension. MMWR Morb Mortal Wkly Rep. 2016 Nov 18;65(45):1261-1264. doi: 10.15585/mmwr.mm6545a3.

2. BEST and TAYLOR - -Physiological Basis of Medical Practice: 155 WILLIAMS and WILKINS COMPANY BALTIMORE 1950.

3. WILLIAMS G.H. et BRAUNWALD E. -Hypertension artérielle- Principes de Médecine Interne. T.R. Harrison: 196: 1024 Médecine-Sciences FLAMMARION PARIS 1989.

4.ACC/AHA/AAPA/ABC/ACPM/AGS/APhA/ASH/ASPC/NMA/PCNA. 2017 Guideline for the Prevention, Detection, Evaluation, and Management of High Blood Pressure in Adults. Report of the American College of Cardiology/American Heart Association Task Force on Clinical Practice Guidelines. Journal of the American college of cardiology vol. 71, no. 19, 2018.

18

Coronary Disease and Heart Infarct

1. ABBOTT R.D., WILSON P.W.F., KANNEL W.B., CASTELLI W.P. -High-Density Lipoprotein Cholesterol, Total Cholesterol Screening, and Myocardial Infarction -The Framingham Study: Arteriosclerosis, 8: 207-211, 1988.

2. LESSER M.A. -Testosterone Propionate Therapy in One Hundred Cases of Angina Pectoris: J. Clin. Endocrinol., 6: 549-557, 1946.

3. MOLLER J. and Einfeldt - Testosterone Treatment of Cardiovascular Diseases SPRINGER-VERLAG BERLIN HEIDELBERG NEW YORK TOKYO 1984.

4. MOLLER J. - Cholesterol SPRINGER-VERLAG BERLIN HEIDELBERG NEW YORK LONDON PARIS TOKYO 1987.

5. KRIEG M., SMITH K., and BARTSCH W. -Demonstration of a Specific Androgen Receptor in Rat Heart Muscle: Relationship between Binding Metabolism and Tissue Levels of Androgens: Endocrinology, 103: 1686-1694, 1978.

6. KRIEG M., SMITH K., and ELVERS B. -Androgen Receptor Translocation from Cytosol of Rat Heart Muscle, Bulbocavernosus Levator Ani Muscle and Prostate into heart Muscle Nuclei: J. Steroid Biochem., 13: 577-587, 1980.

7. BLASIUS R., KAFER K., SEITZ W. - Untersuchungen über die Wirkung von Testosteron auf die Contractilen Strukturproteine des Herzens. Klin. Woch., 34, 11/12, 324, 1956.

8. DOMINIQUE SIMON, MARIE-ALINE CHARLES, KHALIL NAHOUL, GENEVIEVE ORSSAUD, JACQUELINE KREJNSKI, VERONIQUE HULLY, EVELYNE JOUBERT, LAURE PAPOZ, AND EVELINE ESCHWEGE. Association between Plasma Total Testosterone and Cardiovascular Risk Factors in Healthy Adult Men: The Telecom Study. Clin. Endocrinol. Metab., 82: 682-685, 1997.

9. KATYA B. RUBINOW, TOMAS VAISAR, CHONGREN TANG, ALVIN M. MATSUMOTO, JAY W. HEINECKE, AND STEPHANIE T. PAGE. Testosterone replacement in hypogonadal men alters the HDL proteome but not HDL cholesterol efflux capacity'" *J. Lipid Res.* 53: 1376-1383, 2012

10. CHEN Y, FU L, HAN Y, TENG Y, SUN J, XIE R, CAO J. Testosterone replacement therapy promotes angiogenesis after acute myocardial infarction by enhancing the expression of cytokines HIF-1a, SDF-1a, and VEGF. Eur J Pharmacol. 5; 684(1-3):116-24. 2012 Jun.

19

Stiffnesses, Limitation of the Movements, Slipped Discs, and Degenerative Joint Diseases

1. VERZAR F. -Ageing of Connective Tissue: Gerontol., 1: 363-378, 1957.

2. VERZAR F. -Studies on Adaptation as a Method of Gerontological Research, in Ciba Colloq. on Ageing, 3: 60-72, 1957.

3. ROBERT L. -Les Horloges Biologiques Nouvelle Bibliothèque Scientifique FLAMMARION 1989.

4. SOBEL H. and MARMORSTON J. -Hormonal Influences Upon Connective Tissue Changes of Ageing, in PINCUS G (ed) Recent Progress in Hormone Research, vol 14. Academic New York 1958.

5. DEBLED G. Pharmaceutical composition for the prevention of fibrotic diseases. OPRI (Office belge de la propriété intellectuelle) : 100072468. Nº 2019/5905. 13 décembre 2019.

20

Fragile Bones

1. YAN-JIAO WANG, JUN-KUN ZHAN, WU HUANG, YI WANG, YUAN LIU, SHA WANG, PAN TAN, ZHI-YONG TANG, AND YOU-SHUO LIU. Effects of Low-Dose Testosterone Undecanoate Treatment on Bone Mineral Density and Bone Turnover Markers in Elderly Male Osteoporosis with Low Serum Testosterone. Hindawi Publishing Corporation. International Journal of Endocrinology. Volume 2013. Article ID 570413, 6 pages.

21

Skin Wrinkles

1. MARKUS HAAG, TINA HAMANN, ALEXANDRA E. KULLE, FELIX G. RIEPE, THOMAS BLATT, HORST WENCK, PAUL-MARTIN HOLTERHUS, and RETO IVO PEIRANO. Age and skin site-related differences in steroid metabolism in male skin point to a key role of sebocytes in cutaneous hormone metabolism. Dermato-Endocrinology 4 :1, 63-69; January/February/March 2012; ©2012 Landes Bioscience.

23

Metamorphoses of the Silhouette

1. DEBLED G. -L'Hyperoestrogénie Associée à la Dysectasie Fibreuse de l'Urètre Prostatique : Bulletins et Mémoires de la Société de Médecine de Paris, 7 : 199-204, 1980.

24

Kidney Failure

1. DEBLED G. -La Pathologie obstructive Congénitale de l'Uretère Terminal - Thèse d'agrégation de l'enseignement supérieur en Sciences Urologiques, Université Libre de Bruxelles, 18 mai 1971 : Acta Urol. Belg., 39 : 371-465, 1971.

25

Hearing Loss and Vision Troubles

1. DEBLED G. Steroid hormone for the prevention of diseases associated with ageing. (OPRI) Office belge de la propriété intellectuelle: 100072468. Nº 2019/5905. December 13, 2019.

2. DEBLED G : Ageless Woman 2020. HMS WORLD Editions.

3. CURHAN SG, ELIASSEN AH, EAVEY RD, WANG M, LIN BM, CURHAN GC. Menopause and postmenopausal hormone therapy and risk of hearing loss. Menopause. 2017 Sep;24(9):1049-105.

26

Failing Immunity, Aids, Cancers

1. SCHUURS A.H.W.M. and VERHEUL H.A.M. -Effects of Gender and Sex Steroids on the Immune Response: J. Steroid Biochem., 35; 2: 157-172, 1990

2. AHMED S.A., PENHALE W.J. and TALAL N. -Sex Hormones, Immune Responses, and Autoimmune Diseases: AJP -121, 3: 531- 551, 1985.

3. SASSON S. and MAYER M. -Antiglucocorticoid Activity of Androgens in Rat Thymus Lymphocytes: Endocrinology, 108: 760-766, 1981.

4. KLEIN SA, KLAUKE S, DOBMEYER JM, DOBMEYER TS, HELM EB, HOELZER H, ROSSOL R. Substitution of testosterone in an HIV-1 positive patient with hypogonadism and Wasting-syndrome led to a reduced rate of apoptosis. Eur J Med Res. 1997 Jan; 2(1):30-2.

5. RODRIGO T. CALADO, WILLIAM T. YEWDELL, KEISHA L. WILKERSON, JOSHUA A. REGAL, SACHIKO KAJIGAYA, CONSTANTINE A. STRATAKIS, AND NEAL S. YOUNG. Sex hormones, acting on the TERT gene, increase telomerase activity in human primary hematopoietic cells. Blood. 2009 Sep 10; 114 (11): 2236-2243.

6. RUSSEL J. REITER, REMASWAMY SHARMA, DUN-XIAN TAN, RICHARD L. NEEL, FEDOR SIMKO, WALTER MANUCHA, SERGIO ROSALES-CORRALS,

DANIEL P. CARDINALI. Melatonin use for SARS-CoV-2 infection: Time to diversify the treatment portfolio. J Med Virol. 2022;1-3.

7. LAN SH, LEE HZ, CHAO CM, CHANG SP, LU LC, LAI CC. Efficacy of melatonin in the treatment of patients with COVID-19: a systematic review and meta-analysis of randomized controlled trials. J Med Virol. 2022; 94:2102-2107

8. RUSSEL J. REITER, SERGIO A. ROSALES-CORRAL, DUN-XIAN TAN, DARIO ACUNA-CASTROVIEJO, LILAN QIN, SHUN-FA YANG, AND KEXIN XU. Melatonin, a Full-Service Anti-Cancer Agent: Inhibition of Initiation, Progression, and Metastasis. Int J Mol Sci. 2017 Apr; 18(4): 843.

9. DEBLED G. Composition for the treatment of cancers. OPRI (Office belge de la propriété intellectuelle) : 100075876. Nº 2020/5139. March 02 2020.

27

Depression

1. OMS. La dépression. Aide-mémoire Nº 369. Octobre 2012.

2. PERSKY H., SMITH K.D., and BASU G.K. -Relation of Psychologic Measures of Aggression and Hostility to Testosterone Production in Man: Psychosomatic Medicine, 33; 3: 265-277, 1971.

3. SCARAMELLA Th. J. and BROWN W.A. -Serum Testosterone and Aggressiveness in Hockey Players: Psychosomatic Medicine, 40; 3: 262-265, 1978.

4. National Centre for Health Statistics -Vital Statistics Report, Final Mortality Statistics, 1982.

5. ROSE R.M., BERNSTEIN I.S., and GORDON Th. P. -Consequences of Social Conflict on Plasma Testosterone Levels in Rhesus Monkeys: Psychosomatic Medicine, 37; 1: 50-60, 1975.

6. EHRENKRANZ J., BLISS E., and SHEARD M.H. -Plasma Testosterone: Correlation with Aggressive Behaviour and Social Dominance in Man: Psychosomatic Medicine, 36; 6: 469-475, 1974.

7. MAZUR A. and LAMB Th. A. -Testosterone, Status, and Mood in Human Males: Hormones and Behaviour, I4: 236-246, 1980.8

8. LEDERER J. -Le traitement des déviations sexuelles par l'acétate de cyprotérone. Le cerveau et les hormones : 249-260, 1974, dans: L'inhibition pharmacologique de la libido : thérapeutique ou répression ? par SERVAIS J.F. -Acta psychiat. Belg., 82 : 520-546, 1982.

9. de LIGNIERES et MAUVAIS-JARVIS -Endocrinologie de la Dépression. Rôle du Cortisol et des Hormones Sexuelles : Ann. Biol. Clin., 37: 49-57, 1979.

10. KLAIBER E.L., BROVERMAN D.M., VOGEL W., KOBAYASHI Y. -The Use of Steroid Hormones in Depression, in Psychotropic action of hormones: 139 SPECTRUM NEW YORK 1976

11. KHERA M, BHATTACHARYA RK, BLICK G, KUSHNER H, NGUYEN D, MINER MM. The effect of testosterone supplementation on depression symptoms in hypogonadal men from the Testim Registry in the US (TRiUS). Ageing Male. Mar; 15(1):14-21. 2012

12. XIAOWEI Z, ZHENHUA L, YEQING Y, WENJUN B, XIAO FENG W, HUAN S, YONGPING Z. Testosterone therapy improves psychological distress and health-related quality of life in Chinese men with symptomatic late-onset hypogonadism patients. Chin Med J (Engl). 2012 Nov; 125(21):3806-10.

13. KENNETH A. BONNET AND RICHARD P. BROWN in The Biological Role of Dehydroepiandrosterone (DHEA). Walter de Gruyter, Berlin, New York, 1990. p.66-79.

14. JACQUES YOUNG, BEATRICE COUZINET, KHALIL NAHOUL, SYLVIE BRAILLY, PHILIPPE CHANSON, ETIENNE EMILE BAULIEU, AND GILBERT SCHAISON Panhypopituitarism as a Model to Study the Metabolism of Dehydroepiandrosterone (DHEA) in Humans. Journal of Clinical Endocrinology and Metabolism. 82: 2578-2585, 1997

15. R. MORAGA-AMARO, A. VAN WAARDE, J. DOORDUIN, AND E. F. J. DE VRIES. Sex steroid hormones and brain function: PET imageing as a tool for research. J Neuroendocrinol. 2018 Feb; 30(2): e12565.

28

Parkinson's Disease

1. Langston W., PALFREMAN J. The Case of the Frozen Addicts: How the Solution of an Extraordinary Medical Mystery Spawned a Revolution in the Understanding and Treatment of Parkinson's disease. Pantheon Books, New York, 1995.

2. DEBLED G. Steroid hormone for the prevention of diseases associated with ageing. (OPRI) Office belge de la propriété intellectuelle: 100072468. Nº 2019/5905. Decembre 13, 2019.

3. KLAIBER E.L., BROVERMAN D.M., VOGEL W., KOBAYASHI Y. The use of steroid hormones in depression. In Psychotropic action of hormones. Proceedings of the World Congress of biological psychiatry. Buenos Aires. Argentina, September 1974. Spectrum publications INC.

4. Alan L Kaplan, Jim C Hu, Abraham Morgentaler, John P Mulhall, Claude C Schulman, Francesco Montorsi. Testosterone Therapy in Men With Prostate Cancer. Eur. Urol. 2016 May; 69(5): 894–903.

5. A. Yassin, K. AlRumaihi, R. Alzubaidi, S. Alkadhi & A. Al Ansari. Testosterone, testosterone therapy, and prostate cancer. The Ageing Male 2019, 22:4, 219-227.

6. DEBLED G. Composition for the treatment of cancers. OPRI (Office belge de la propriété intellectuelle) : 100075876. Nº 2020/5139. March 02 2020.

29

Dementias and Alzheimer's Disease

1. Lilly. Press Release Archives. Lilly Announces Top-Line Results of Solanezumab Phase 3 Clinical Trial. Nov 23, 2016.

2. DEBLED G. Steroid hormone for the prevention of diseases associated with ageing. (OPRI) Office belge de la propriété intellectuelle: 100072468. Nº 2019/5905. December 13, 2019.

3. Alzheimer's Association, 2019. Alzheimer's Disease Facts and Figures.

4. RASHAD HUSSAIN, ABDEL M. GHOUMARI, BARTOSZ BIELECKI, JÉRÔME STEIBEL, NELLY BOEHM, PHILIPPE LIERE, WENDY B. MACKLIN, NARENDER KUMAR, RENÉ HABERT, SAKI NA MHAOUTY-KODJA, FRANÇOIS TRONCHE, REGINE SITRUK-WARE, MICHAEL SCHUMACHER, AND M. SAID GHANDOUR. The neural androgen receptor: a therapeutic target for myelin repair in chronic demyelination. Brain: 136; 132- 146. May 2013.

5. Dementia. A public Health Priority. WHO report 2012.

6. W. SUE T GRIFFIN, Ph.D. and STEVEN W BARGER, Ph.D. Neuroinflammatory Cytokines-The Common Thread in Alzheimer's Pathogenesis *US Neurol.* 2010: 6(2): 19-27.

7. W. SUE T. GRIFFIN, PH.D. Neuroinflammatory Cytokine Signaling, and Alzheimer's Disease. N Engl J Med 2013; 368:770-771February 21, 2013

8. VOM BERG J, PROKOP S, MILLER KR, OBST J, KÄLIN RE, LOPATEGUI-CABEZAS I, WEGNER A, MAIR F, SCHIPKE CG, PETERS O, WINTERY, BECHER B, HEPPNER FL. Inhibition of IL-12/IL-23 signaling reduces Alzheimer's disease-like pathology and cognitive decline. Nat Med. 2012 Dec; 18(12): 1812-9.doi: 10.1038/nm.2965. Epub 2012 Nov 25.

9. GUNNAR K. GOURAS, HUAXI XU, RACHEL S. GROSS, JEFFREY P. GREENFIELD, BING HAI, RONG WANG, AND PAUL GREENGARD. Testosterone reduces the neuronal secretion of Alzheimer's β-amyloid peptides. Proc Nati Acad Sci U S A. 2000 February 1; 97(3): 1202–1205.

10. GANDY S, ALMEIDA OP, FONTE J, LIM D, WATERRUS A, SPRY N, FLICKER L, MARTINS RN. Chemical andropause and amyloid-beta peptide. JAMA. 2001 May 2; 285(17):2195-6.

11. EMILY R. ROSARIO, Neuroscience Graduate Program, MS. Lilly Chang, MD. Frank Z. Stanczyk, Ph.D. CHRISTIAN J. PIKE, P. Age-Related Testosterone Depletion and the Development of Alzheimer Disease *JAMA. 2004; 292(12):1431-1432.*

12. EMILY R. ROSARIO AND CHRISTIAN J. PIKE. Brain Research Reviews 57, Issue 2, 14 March 2008, Pages 44-453.

13. ROSARIO ER, CHANG L, HEAD EH, STANCZYK FZ, PIKE CJ. Brain levels of sex steroid hormones in men and women during normal ageing and in Alzheimer's disease Neurobiol Ageing. 2011 Apr ;32(4) :604-13. Epub 2009 May 9.

14. BRADFORD T. WINSLOW, MD, MARY K. ONYSKO, Pharm. D, CHRISTIAN M. STOB, DO, KATHLEEN A. HAZLEWOOD. *Treatment of Alzheimer's Disease.* Am Fam Physician. 2011 Jun 15; 83(12):1403-1412.

15. HIDETAKA OTA, MASAHIRO AKISHITA, TAKUYU AKIYOSHI, TOMOAKI KAHYO, M. ITSUTOSHI SETOU, SUMITO OGAWA, KATSUYA LIJIMA, MASATO ETO, YASUYOSHI OUCHI. Testosterone Deficiency Accelerates Neuronal and Vascular Ageing of SAMP8 Mice: Protective Role of eNOS and SIRT1. PLoS ONE I www.plosone.org January 2012 - Volume 7 - Issue 1 - e29598.

16. CHI-FAI LAU, YUEN-SHAN HO, CLARA HIU-LING HUNG, SUTHICHA WUWONGSE, CHUN-HEI POON, KIN CHIU, XIFEI YANG, LEUNG-WING CHU, AND RAYMOND CHUEN-CHUNG CHANG. Protective Effects of Testosterone on Presynaptic Terminals against Oligomeric β-Amyloid Peptide in Primary Culture of Hippocampal Neurons. Hindawi Publishing Corporation. BioMed Research International. Volume 2014, Article ID 103906, 12 pages. http://dx.doi.org/10.1155/2014/103906.

30

Stroke

1. CDC, NCHS. Underlying Cause of Death 1999-2013 on CDCWONDEROnline Database2015; e29-322.
http: Uwonder.cdc.govlycd-jcd10.html, released 2015. Data are from the Multiple Cause of Death Files, 1999-2013, as compiled from data provided by the 57 vital statistics jurisdictions through theVital Statistics Cooperative Program. Accessed Feb. 3, 2015.

2. KATHLEEN STRONG CM. RUTH BONITA. Preventing stroke: saving lives around the world. *Lancet Neurol,* vol.6, №2, 2007, p.182-87.

3. MOZAFFARIAN D, BENJAMIN EJ, GO AS, ET AL. Heart disease and stroke statistics-2015 update: a report from the American Heart Association. *Circulation. 2015; e 29-322.*

33

Hormonal Treatment

1. MEEKER AK, SOMMERFELD HJ, COFFEY DS. Telomerase is activated in the prostate and seminal vesicles of the castrated rat. Endocrinology. 1996 Dec; 137(12):5743-6.

2. DEBLED G. Composition for the treatment of cancer. Office belge de la propriété intellectuelle (OPRI) : 100075876. № 2020/5139. 02 mars 2020.

3. MINDY KIM GRAHAM AND ALAN MEEKER. Telomeres and telomerase in prostate cancer development and therapy. nat rev urol. 2017 october ; 14(10) : 607–619.

4. DEBLED G. The menopausal disease. Approaches to ageing control: 19:17-24, October 2015.

5. DEBLED G. Mesterolone pharmaceutical composition for dihydrotestosterone deficiencies in the woman. EPO. Application Patent N° 121/6851.9 - 1466/268/215 European Patent Bulletin 18/48 of 28.11.18.

6. DEBLED G. The androgenic disease of andropause. SEMAL congress, Seville, October 5, 2019.

7. DEBLED G. Steroid hormone for the prevention of diseases associated with ageing. (OPRI) Office belge de la propriété intellectuelle: 100072468. № 2019/5905. December 13, 2019.

8. BASARIA S, COVIELLO AD, TRAVISON TG, et al. Adverse events associated with testosterone administration. N Engl J Med. 2010; 363(2):109-122.

9. MØLLER J. and Einfeldt - Testosterone Treatment of Cardiovascular Diseases. SPRINGER-VERLAG. BERLIN.

10. G. DEBLED. Androgernic disease in men. HMS World, 2026.

11. GOOREN L.J.G. -Long-Term Safety of the Oral Androgen Testosterone Undecanoate: Int. J. Androl., 9: 21-26, 1986.

12. FENELEY MR, CARRUTHERS M. Is Testosterone Treatment Good for the Prostate? Study of Safety during Long-Term Treatment. J Sex Med. 2012 Jun 6.

13. MOLLY M. SHORES, NICHOLAS L. SMITH, CHRISTOPHER W. FORSBERG, BRADLEY D. ANAWALT, AND ALVIN M. MATSUMOTO. Testosterone Treatment and Mortality in Men with Low Testosterone Levels. J. Clin. Endocrinol. Metab. 97: 2050-2058. 2012.

14. DEBLED G. The male climacteric prime cause of sex involution. The Tenth annual international symposium on man and his environment in health and disease. February 27-March 1, 1992. Dallas. Texas. The U.S.A.

15. DEBLED G. The male climacteric prime cause of ageing. The Tenth annual international symposium on man and his environment in health and disease. February 27-March 1, 1992. Dallas. Texas. The U.S.A.

16. DEBLED G. Androgenic disease in Men. HMS World Editions. 2025

17.   https://resources.bayer.com.au/resources/uploads/PI/file9420.pdf (2007-2009).

18. Christine P. Nguyen, M.D., Mark S. Hirsch, M.D., David Moeny, R.Ph., M.P.H., Suresh Kaul, M.D., M.P.H., Mohamed Mohamoud, Pharm.D., M.P.H., Hylton V. Joffe, M.D., M.M.Sc. Testosterone and "Age-Related Hypogonadism" — FDA Concerns. N Engl J Med. 2015 Aug 20;373(8):689-91. doi: 10.1056/NEJMp1506632.

https://www.ncbi.nlm.nih.gov/pmc/articles/PMC8905399/

19. DEBLED G. Adverse effects of 5-alpha-reductase inhibitors. SEMAL: 2nd International congress anti-ageing medicine. Miami, February 6th to 9th,2020

20. DEBLED G. Ageless Woman. HMS WORLD Editions, 2020

21. DEBLED G. Course: The Androgenic Disease of Andropause and Menopause. SEMAL. III Congreso Intercontinental de Medicina Antienvejecimiento. Hotel Hilton. Panamá 17 de marzo 2022, (In Spanish).

22. DEBLED G. The Androgenic Disease of Menopause. SEMAL. III Congreso Intercontinental de Medicina Antienvejecimiento. Hotel Hilton. Panamá 19 de marzo 2022, (In Spanish).

23. DEBLED G. The Prevention of Prostate Adenoma. SEMAL. III Congreso Intercontinental de Medicina Antienvejecimiento. Hotel Hilton. Panamá 17-18 de marzo 2022, (In Spanish).

24. DEBLED G. Androgenic disease. Etiology and biochemistry. IVth Intercontinental Congress of Anti-Ageing Medicine and Medical Aesthetics. Bogota, February 29 to March 2, 2024.[*]

25. DEBLED G. Androgenic disease. Management of hormonal treatment. IV Intercontinental Congress of Anti-Ageing Medicine and Medical Aesthetics. Bogota, February 29 - March 2, 2024.[*]

26. DEBLED G : The Androgenic Disease in Men. HMS WORLD, 2025

27. DEBLED G. Prostate Ageing Control. HMS WORLD Editions, 2026

---

[*]Androgenic Disease in Men, explains the principles of androgenic disease and covers the management details of the preventive treatment of ageing diseases.

www.ingramcontent.com/pod-product-compliance
Lightning Source LLC
Chambersburg PA
CBHW070223190526
45169CB00001B/64